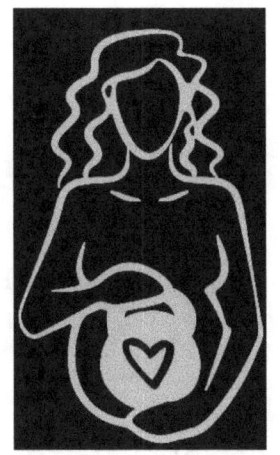

FIT & EXPECTING

A Better Shape of YOU

WILLIAM RAMON

WILLIAM RAMON

Copyright © 2019 William Ramon

All Rights Reserved

ISBN: 978-1-0824-7204-6

This book is dedicated to ALL the resilient mothers and female bosses who lead by example day in and day out! I am so happy and grateful for all the strong female figures in my life. THANK YOU!

I also dedicate this book to everyone who has had the courage to look inward and embrace your true self!

CONTENTS

FIT & EXPECTING

FIT & EXPECTING

FIT & EXPECTING

FIT & EXPECTING

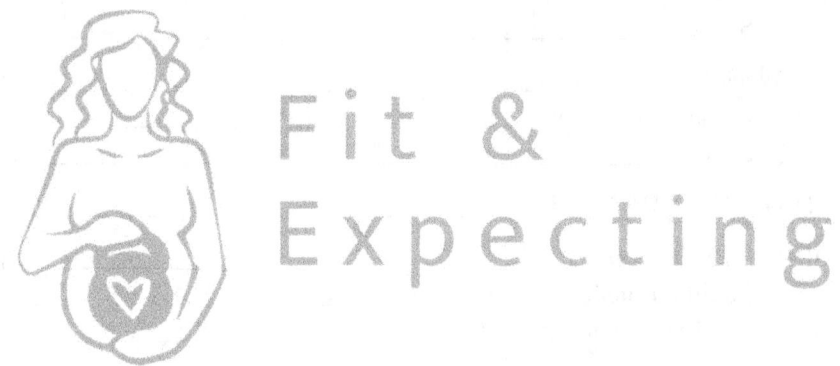

FOREWORD

Hey Mama,

Twelve years ago, I was working at East Bank Club, one of the largest health clubs in the world, and I stumbled on a prenatal fitness certification. I was thirty-six years old and had no children, but I was fascinated with all things fitness so I decided to sign up.

I learned more about the female body than I had ever known existed and quickly understood the massive benefits of exercising throughout pregnancy and even after pregnancy.

Two years later, I was pregnant myself. Whoa...! Whole new ballgame. I was not expecting the epic changes that were happening in my body. And exercising through my own pregnancy was definitely an adventure. I tried my best to apply what I'd learned, and I had a great experience being pregnant.

Although every pregnancy is so unique, there are common things we can all do to make our pregnancy the fittest and healthiest pregnancy possible. But most of them remain a mystery.

What I was craving was a plan. A solid plan for exactly what I should do, week by week. I longed for it. I even reached out to the instructors from my prenatal fitness cert and asked if they had more custom workouts for women to follow. They didn't. I was left high and dry.

I'm happy to say I had two happy, healthy, all-natural labors and delivered two happy, healthy kids, thanks in large part to exercising through my pregnancy, even without a plan.

Last year, I met William Ramon at a book-writing retreat in New York. When he told me about his passion for prenatal fitness, I was really excited—not for myself (no more kids over here!), but for all the women whose lives he will touch.

And then this book was born. It's everything I wished I'd had and more. This book is a gem. It can and will change your life. If you follow his advice and apply all you learn, you'll sail through to the other side of your pregnancy and thrive afterward.

You might even name your first-born William!

Wishing you the happiest, healthiest pregnancy possible.

You're already an amazing mom!

Steffani LeFevour
Bestselling author of *You Are A Badass Mom*
Happiness Coach, Mindset Mentor
Badass Mom to two badass kids

I.

Pre-Pregnancy and Postpartum Fitness Preparation

WILLIAM RAMON

INTRODUCTION

GROWING UP, I WAS not only the emotional middle child, but I was the only boy of three siblings, sandwiched between my 2 sisters! Both of my grandmas, Olivia and Gloria, played a major role in raising me. The unconditional love they displayed for their family through their actions was palpable, endearing, and infectious. Most of what I learned and how I was raised growing up was influenced heavily by women.

Although my dad was in the picture, he worked day in and day out, building a business to provide the best opportunities for us, and therefore wasn't around much. When I started middle school, my dad began to get serious about the woman who would later become my stepmom. She had two children of her own, one boy and one girl. I finally had a brother—*ha!*

As a kid, I can recall quite vividly my mom's and grandmothers' love for children. They were constantly reliving the day we were all born, often telling us the same few stories in a different manner or context, over and over again.

Each time a significant storm rolled through our area, the story was told about how I was born on a gloomy day and usually ended with their expressed excitement about the day when I finally give them a grandchild!

As my Grandma Olivia grew ill, just before her passing, she started to have audio-visual hallucinations. When I visited her, she would always speak about the children in the room, although there were no actual children staying with her. She would also always speak proudly about the four grandchildren and five great-grandchildren she had helped raise. Her family, her children, her babies—this was her life's work and devotion.

I am so happy and grateful for the women who brought me up. Mothers, Godmothers, grandmothers, and great-grandmothers alike play such a pivotal part in our upbringing!

Helping mothers is my labor of love! Through this text, I hope to inspire, create awareness, educate, and help mothers be the strongest version of themselves—not only physically, but energetically and mentally, as well.

PREFACE

LIFT FOR LONGEVITY

PREGNANCY DOESN'T HAVE to be any sort of a setback whatsoever! It is the most special nine months a woman can possibly experience! Being fit during your pregnancy gives you a great advantage.

Then, continuing to train once the baby is born is even *more* important! With postpartum depression affecting so many moms today, preventative and therapeutic methods such as exercise can provide tremendous and essential relief.

There are many things women can do not only during pregnancy, but *before* and *after* their pregnancy, to help increase the quality of life for themselves and their soon-to-be newborn! If you're planning on building a family or want to have a child in the near future, start preparing *NOW*!

For those of you who weren't planning on having a child and have already given birth, if you're cleared by your physician for exercise, adopt a strength-training regimen!

Even if you have planned your pregnancy, it is vital and exponentially beneficial to begin lifting weights once you have the green light from your doctor.

I understand not all mothers can exercise immediately after conceiving. For those of you who cannot, start getting mentally prepared before you get cleared. So, when the time is appropriate, you're ready to begin without hesitation.

WHY WOMEN AND MOMS ALIKE SHOULD RESISTANCE TRAIN

THERE IS A VERY COMMON misconception amongst not only my female clients, but many women I have spoken to about their fitness-related goals, that goes like this: I don't want to lift weights too much, because I don't want to look like a guy.

While it is completely understandable why women are concerned about this, *it's a myth!* Although women do have small amounts of testosterone, it is nowhere near enough to develop musculature equivalent to a man. However, the fantastic news is, women who resistance train have a *massive* edge in life. Not only physically, but cognitively, as well!

As we all know, exercise not only benefits our aesthetic appearance, but it enhances our mental faculties, too. In conjunction with being mentally stronger, the quality of life you live will increase.

Physiologically, the more muscle we build through lifting weights, the more calories we burn while we are not exerting ourselves or exercising. This alone will help you maintain a healthy weight and combat an inability to keep unwanted weight off.

In our day-to-day life, when we are stronger, we are typically happier. Most of you are thinking, "What is this guy talking about?" What I mean, simply, is your daily parental tasks become much more seamless.

Laundry baskets, all of a sudden, get lighter. Holding the baby on your strong side and the diaper bag or many other necessary items on the other side seems routine: light to no work, so to speak.

Being a mother requires a lot of time and energy. It's inevitable, but each of us WILL get stressed out. Having an outlet, such as working out, is a saving grace! It is that one hour or so we all have, two to three times a week, that can really help us reset and focus on ourselves. Then you, the mother of the family, can maintain a healthy life balance.

As you begin to read this book and execute the workouts, please memorize the quote below and keep it in mind as you evolve in each phase of the program!

"Self-comparison is the thief of joy."

You are reading this book and implementing the strategies for the betterment of yourself first! Who cares what Mrs. Jones weighs? What size jeans she wears? Or even how she looks in a bikini? That is all irrelevant. Of course, we all want to look a certain way, but you shouldn't ever want to look like anyone but yourself!

You have it all. You are perfect the way you are, as you work steadfastly to get where you want to be. This is all about self-growth, challenging yourself to be better than you used to be. It is about taking care of yourself first, which in turn allows you to be there for your colleagues, family, friends, and loved ones alike.

With that being said, commit to yourself! Follow the program as closely as possible, and stay true to discipline. Be present during each session, and realize that all of this is a day-at-a-time process. All we have control over is this very moment in time and the decisions we make in it; maximize it, envelop yourself in it, and experience true growth, as a result!

CHAPTER 1

TRAINING OVERVIEW

FOR THE NEXT nine months, we will have three scheduled workouts per week. That is a total of thirty-six weeks and 108 full-body workouts. These training sessions will not only burn fat, but they will help you build muscle and increase your overall strength and mobility.

Throughout these 108 workouts, you will become familiar with over 100 total exercises and dynamic warm-up drills, all of which are illustrated for you via photo!

Each workout will consist of exercises that target every muscle group, maximizing not only your time but the number of calories you burn overall!

Before beginning every session, each person is required to complete a dynamic warm-up, which is also a form of corrective exercise.

Corrective exercise teaches you how to move with the correct muscles, optimizing your fluid joint movement. With a conscious focus on joint alignment and range of motion, the likelihood for future injuries, nagging aches, and pains decreases.

Dynamic warm-ups also allow you to prepare the central nervous system for exercise, which in turn helps provide sufficient blood flow to the area being targeted during the warm-up. These warm-ups can also be a very effective way to start your day, providing added energy to the individual!

Corrective exercise is so vital for each and every person. The lifestyle most us live is characterized by long periods of sitting, lying down, or even standing up. This behavior makes it difficult for us to move to the best of our ability.

WILLIAM RAMON

II.

First Trimester Fitness Program

WILLIAM RAMON

CHAPTER 2

MONTHS 1-3

THE FOCUS OF THE first three months in this program is broken down into three simple main points:

1.) **Acclamation:** Getting acclimated to not only the workouts and soreness, but learning the vernacular of the program and understanding *why* we are performing the exercise. This is imperative. When we understand and state our *why*, confidence increases as a byproduct.

2.) **Consistency:** Showing up, week after week, session after session, is a non-negotiable when it comes to success within any program we begin. While it is completely understandable to have off days and family emergencies, those occurrences *do not* define you as a whole. Remember why you are doing this program: to help you regain focus. This program is conquered one day at a time! Everyone who is successful with this program has achieved their best by taking action one day at a time. Consistency is KING—well, in your case, QUEEN! Ha!

3.) **Patience:** During not only this program, but throughout life in general, we must deploy patience! Patience with ourselves, with the work it takes, and with the consistency it demands. We must be patient as we execute the process. Some of the movements may become redundant to some of you, but please remember, engraining the fundamentals is a pre-requisite to success in ANYTHING you do! Trust it! You'll be so happy and grateful you did.

The focus of each workout is to incorporate all major muscle groups each and every single workout, providing balance maximal caloric expenditure.

Recommended Tools for Maximal Results (Months 1-3)

* Minibands
* Foam Roller
* Balance Pad

MONTH #1

WEEKS 1-4

~Week #1~

Dynamic Warm-up:

1. **Thread the needle** @10-15 repetitions each side.
2. **Standing Wall Slides** @10-15 repetitions each side.
3. **High Knee to Heel Kick** @10-15 reps each side.

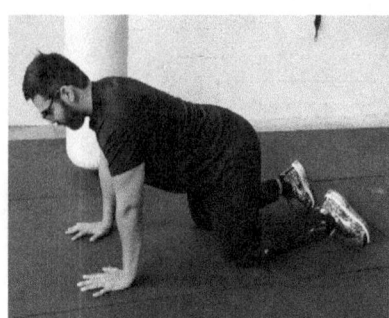 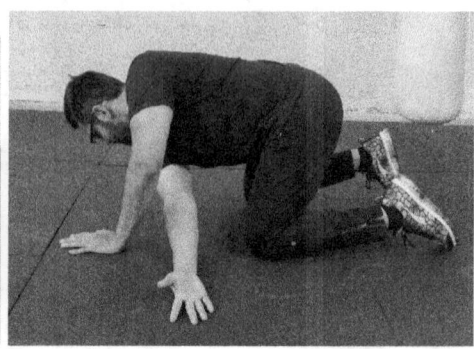

Thread the Needle 1-2

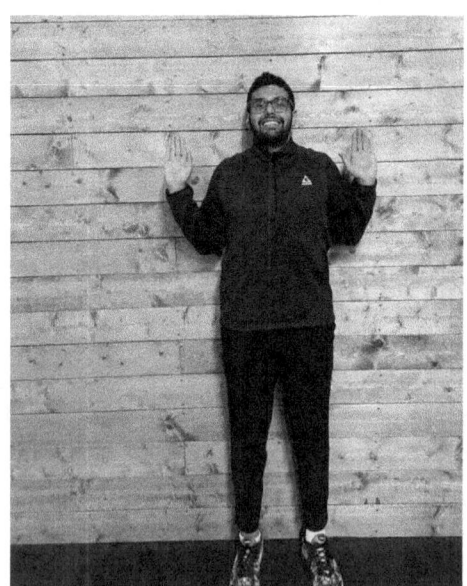 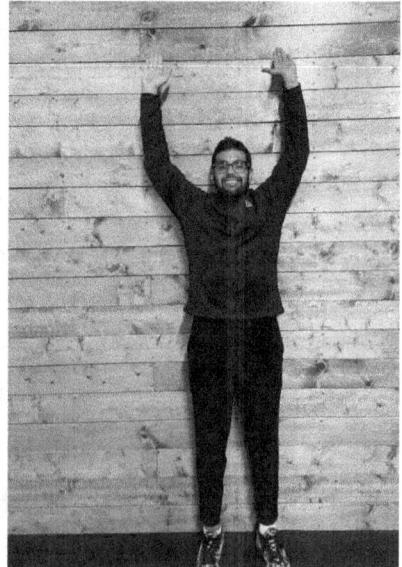

Standing Wall Slides1-2

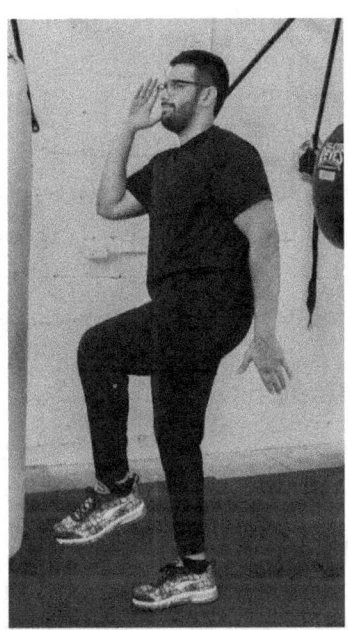

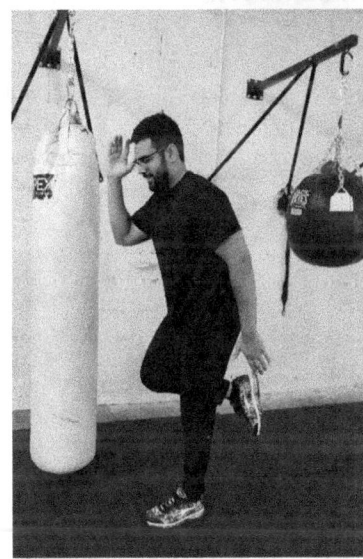 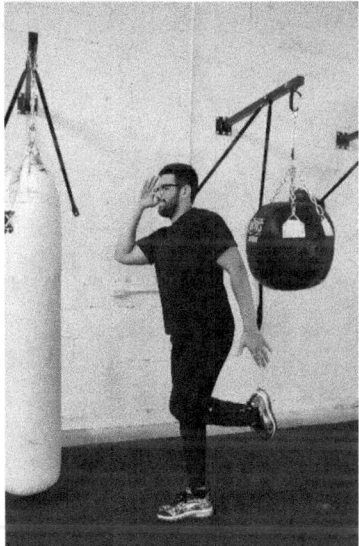

High Knee to Heel Kick 1-3

Session:

1. Air Squat w/**Goblet Setup** @15-20 reps, followed by **Glute Bridge** @15-20 reps.

    Please complete 4 total sets. *Rest* no more than ninety seconds after each set. **Prone Push-up** (use modifications for this movement, if you cannot complete the repetitions with proper form; please refer to modified push-up options in the Movement Photo Archive) @10-15 repetitions, followed by **Standing Band Row (Neutral Grip)** @10-15 repetitions.

    Please complete 4 total sets. *Rest* no more than sixty seconds after each set.

2. **Dumbbell Loaded Carry (Neutral Grip)** @30-45 seconds, followed by a **bracing plank** @15-20 seconds (modify if necessary; please refer to modified bracing plank in the Movement Photo Archive.)

    Please complete 4 total sets. *Rest* no more than sixty seconds after each set.

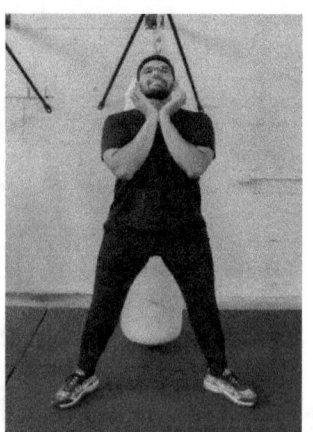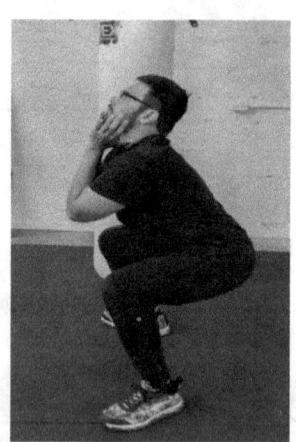

Goblet setup Bodyweight 1-2

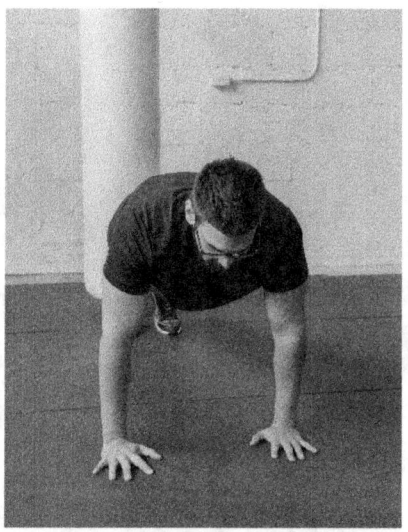

Prone Push-up

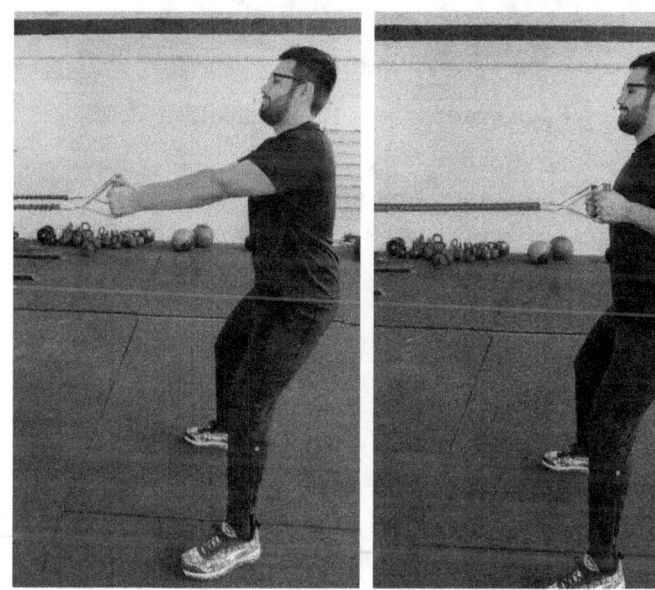

Standing Band Row (Neutral Grip)

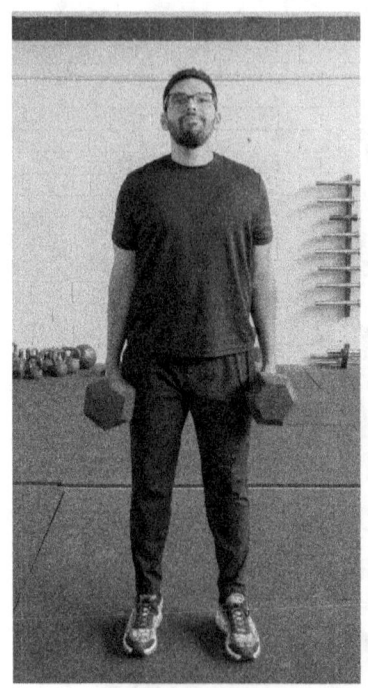 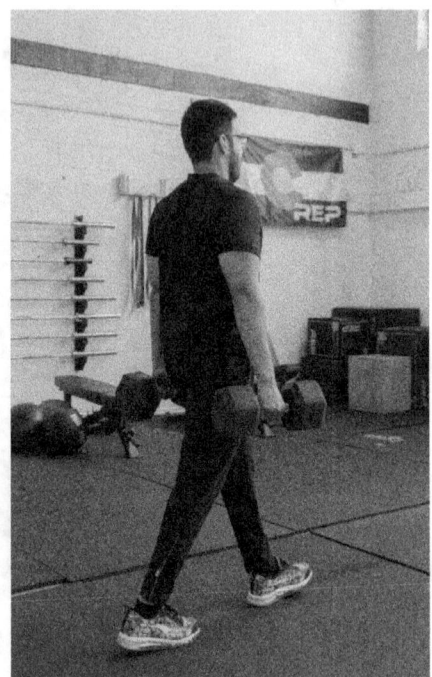

Dumbbell Loaded Carry (Neutral Grip) 1-2

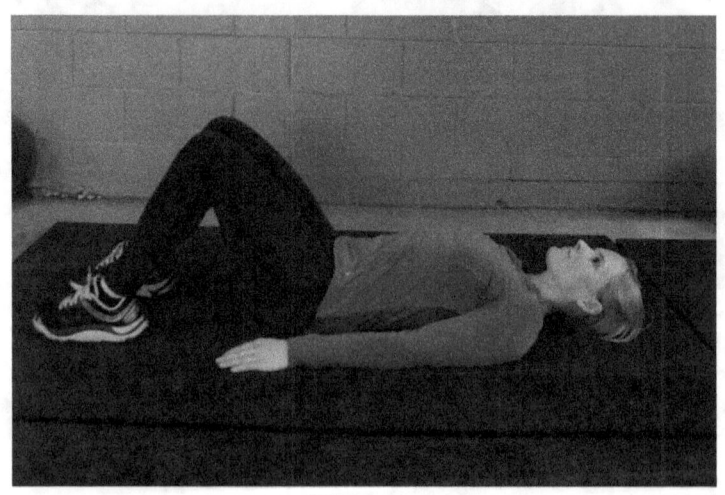

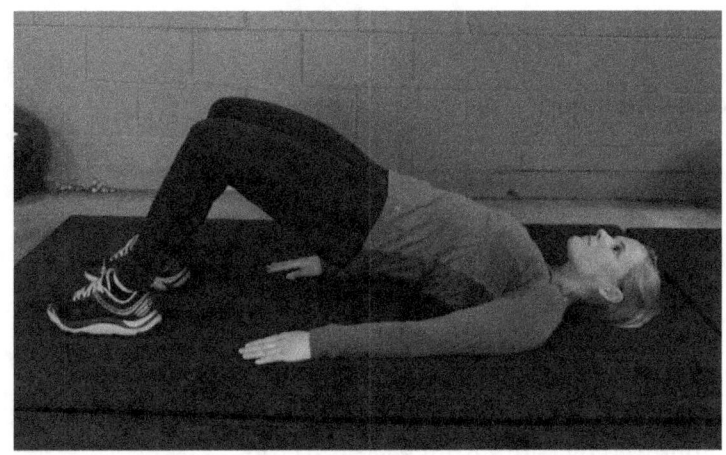

Glute Bridge 1-2

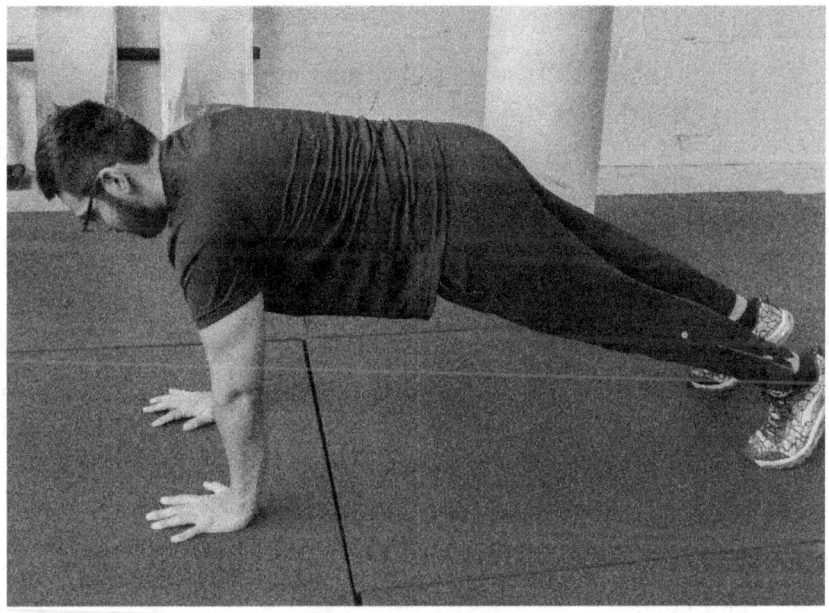

Bracing Plank

Squeeze glutes together to fulfill the bracing requirement of this particular plank

~Week #2~

Dynamic Warm-up:

1. Thread the needle @10-15 repetitions each side.

2. Standing Wall Slides @10-15 repetitions each side.

3. High Knee to Heel Kick @10-15 repetitions each side.

Session:

1. **Dumbbell Goblet Squat w/ Goblet Setup** @15-20 reps, followed by Glute Bridge @15-20 reps

   Please complete 4 total sets. *Rest* no more ninety seconds after each set.

2. Incline Push-up (use modifications for this movement, if you cannot complete the repetitions with proper form; please refer to modified incline push-up options in the Movement Photo Archive) @10-15 repetitions, followed by **Standing Band Row (Pronated to Neutral Grip)** @10-15 repetitions.

   Please complete 4 total sets. *Rest* no more than sixty seconds after each set.

3. **Dumbbell Loaded Carry (Supinated Grip)** @30-45 seconds, followed by a bracing plank @15-20 seconds (modify if necessary; please refer to modified bracing plank in the movement photo archive).

   Please complete 4 total sets. *Rest* no more than sixty seconds after each set.

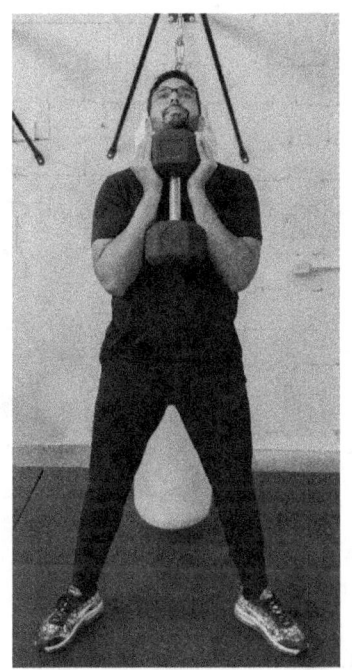
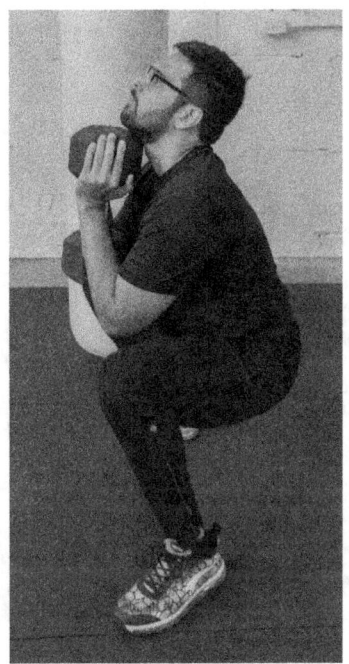

Dumbbell Goblet Squat w/ Goblet Setup 1-2

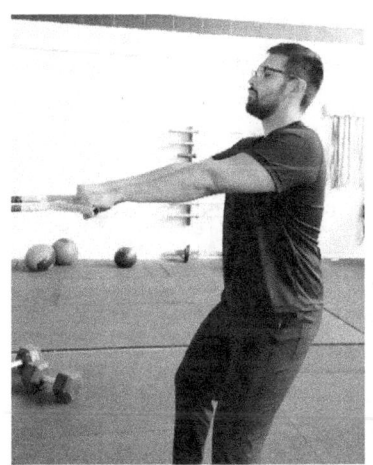
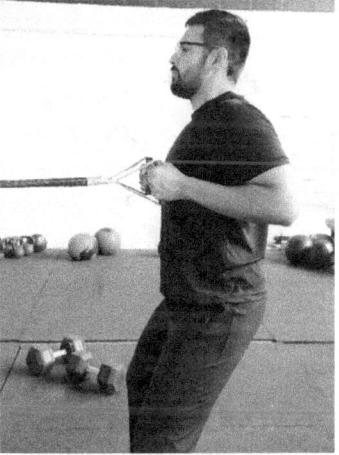

Standing Band Row (Pronated to Neutral Grip) 1-2

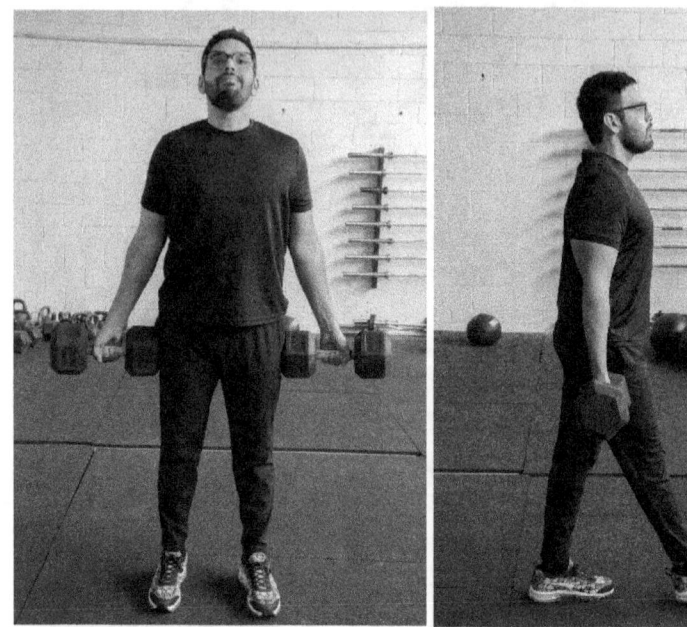

Dumbbell Loaded Carry 1-2

~Week #3~

Dynamic Warm-up:

1. Thread the needle @10-15 repetitions each side.

2. Standing Wall Slides @10-15 repetitions each side.

3. High Knee to Heel Kick @10-15 reps each side.

Session:

1. Dumbbell Goblet Squat w/ Goblet Setup @15-20 reps, followed by **Frog Pump Glute Bridge** @15-20 reps.

Please complete 4 total sets. *Rest* no more than ninety seconds after each set.

2. Prone Push-up (use Modifications for this movement, if you cannot complete the repetitions with proper form; please refer to modified push-up options in the Movement Photo Archive) @10-15 repetitions, followed by **Band Pull-Aparts** @10-15 repetitions

   Please complete 4 total sets. *Rest* no more than sixty seconds after each set.

3. Dumbbell Loaded Carry (Neutral Grip) @30-45 seconds, followed by a bracing plank @15-20 seconds (modify if necessary; please refer to modified bracing plank in the Movement Photo Archive).

   Please complete 4 total sets. *Rest* no more than sixty seconds after each set.

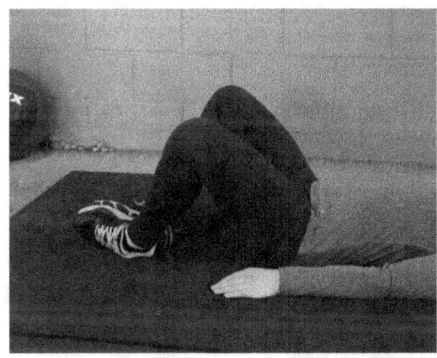 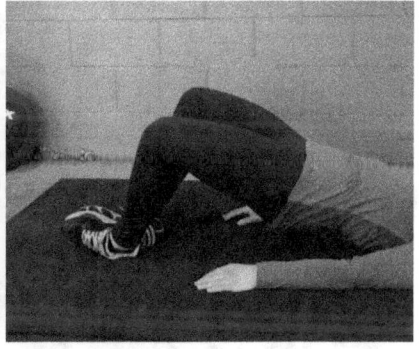

Frog Pump Glute Bridge

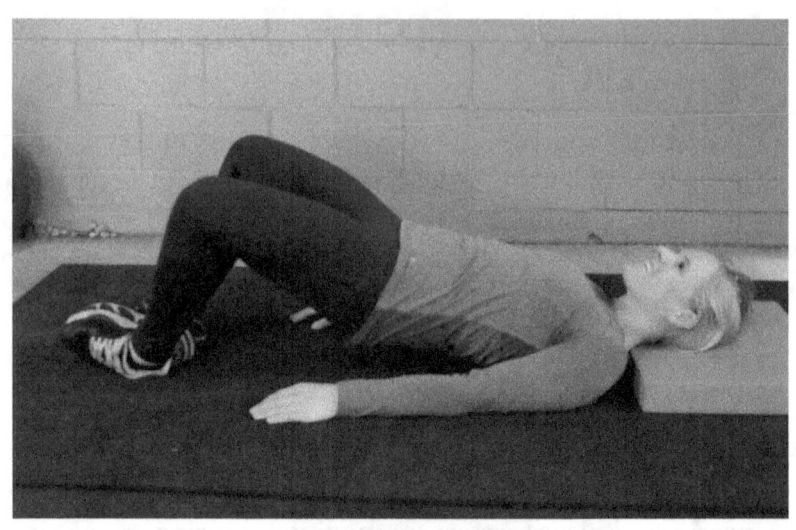

Frog Pump Glute Bridge 3

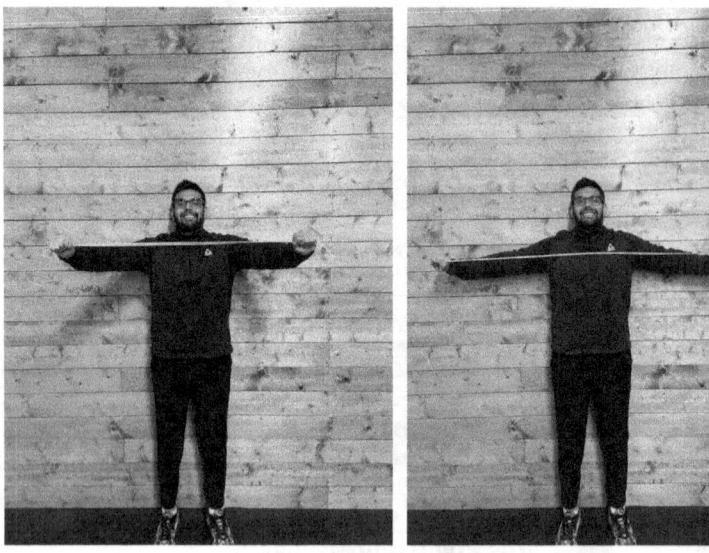

Band Pull-Aparts 1-2

~Week #4~

Dynamic Warm-up:

1. Thread the needle @10-15 repetitions each side.

2. Standing Wall Slides @10-15 repetitions each side.

3. High Knee to Heel Kick @10-15 reps each side.

Session:

1. Air Squat w Goblet Setup @20-25 reps, followed by Glute Bridge @20-25 reps.

    Please complete 4 total sets. REST no more than ninety seconds after each set.

2. Incline Push-up (use modifications for this movement, if you cannot complete the repetitions with proper form; please refer to modified push-up options in the Movement Photo Archive) @10-15 repetitions, followed by Band Pull-Aparts @10-15 repetitions.

    Please complete 4 total sets. REST no more than sixty seconds after each set.

3. Dumbbell Loaded Carry (Neutral Grip) @30-45 seconds, followed by a bracing plank @15-20 seconds (modify if necessary; please refer to modified bracing plank in the Movement Photo Archive).

    Please complete 4 total sets. *Rest* no more than sixty seconds after each set.

MONTH #2

WEEKS 1-4

~Week 1~

Dynamic Warm-up:

1. **Thread the Needle w/ Foam Roller** @10-15 repetitions each side.

2. **Inch Worms** @10 -15 repetitions each side.

3. **Seated Wall Slides** @10-15 reps each side.

Session:

1. **Mini-band Goblet Squat w/ Goblet Setup** @15-20 reps, followed by **DB Deadlifts** @10-15 reps.

Please complete 4 total sets. *Rest* no more than ninety seconds after each set. (Mini-bands are placed above the knee only for the goblet squat.)

2. **Incline Dumbbell Hammer Press** @10-15 repetitions, followed by **Incline DB Row** @10-15 repetitions.

   Please complete 4 total sets. *Rest* no more than sixty seconds after each set.

3. **Marching Dumbbell Loaded Carry (Neutral Grip)** @30-45 seconds, followed by Mountain Climbers @10 each side. (Modify if necessary; please refer to modified Mountain Climber in the Movement Photo Archive.)

   Please complete 4 total sets. *Rest* no more than ninety seconds after each set.

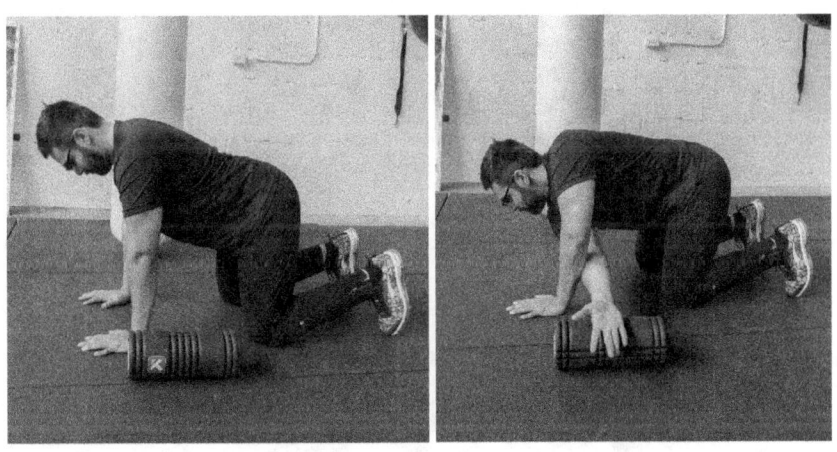

Thread the needle w/ Roller Start

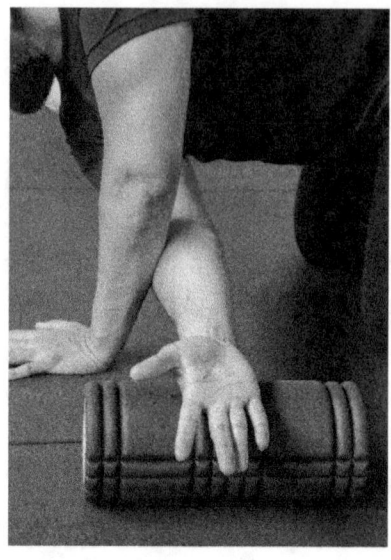

Thread the Needle w/ Foam Roller 1-3

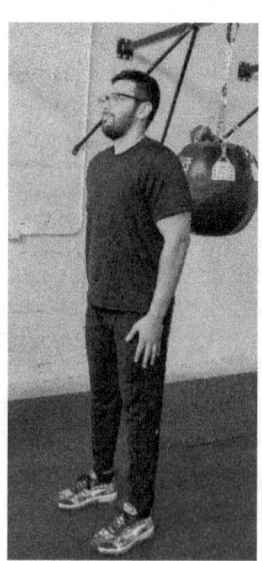
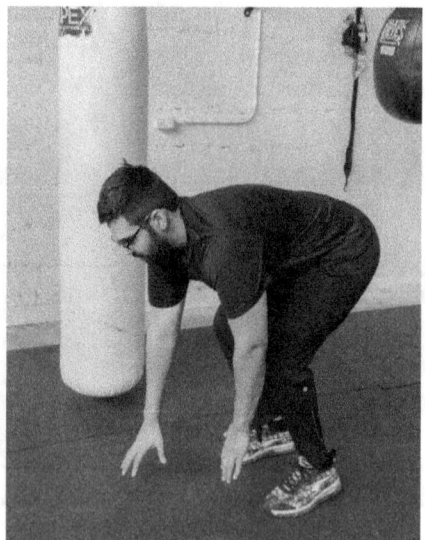

Inch Worm Start

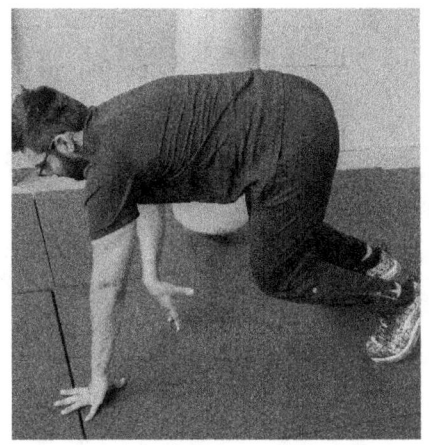
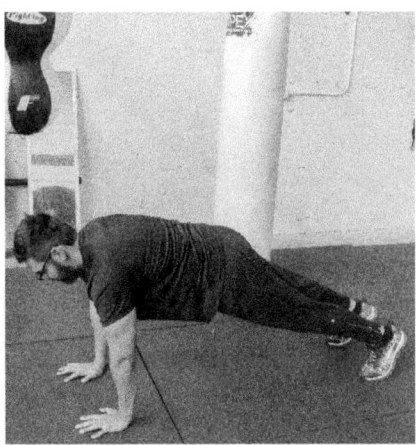

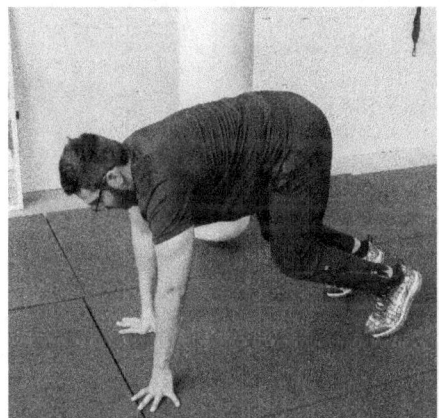
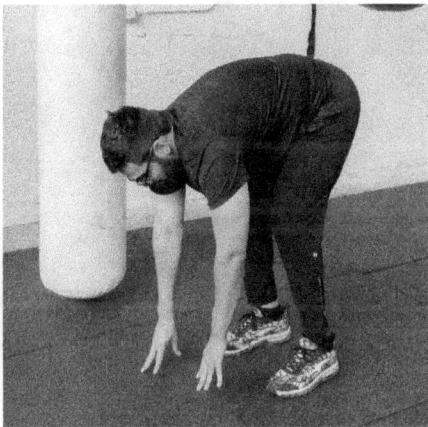

Inch Worm 1-6

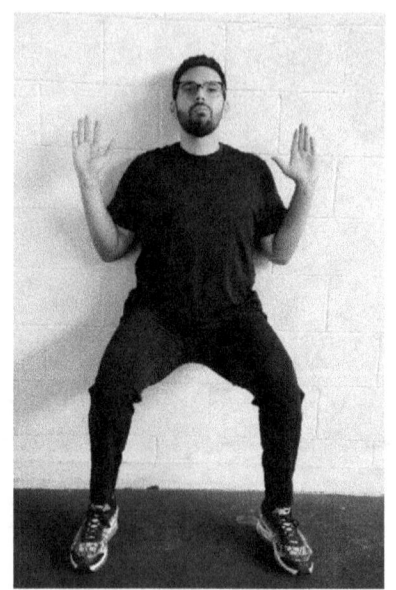 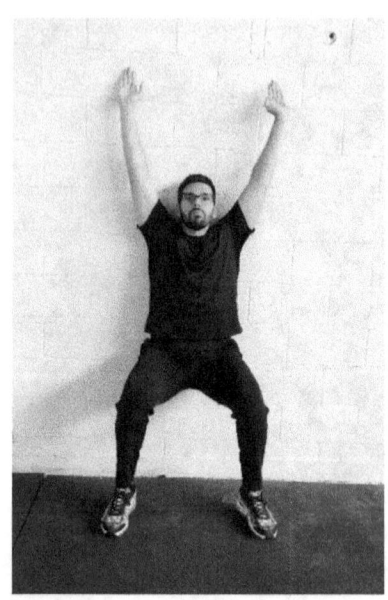

Seated Wall Slides 1-2

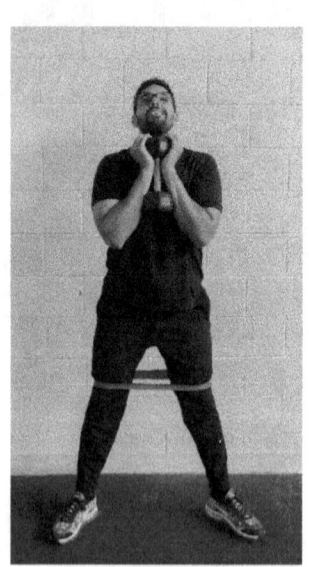 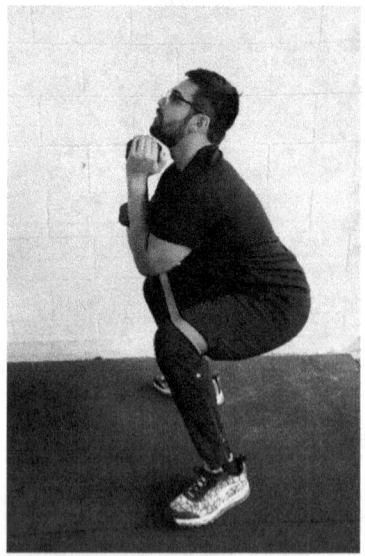

Mini-band Goblet Squat w/ Goblet Setup

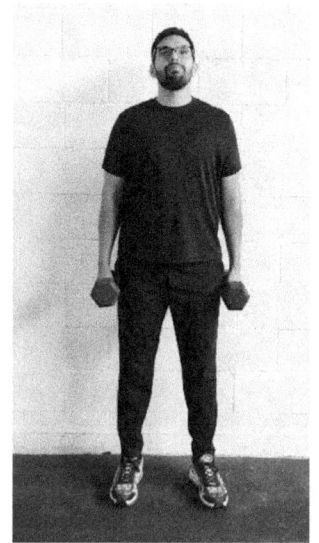 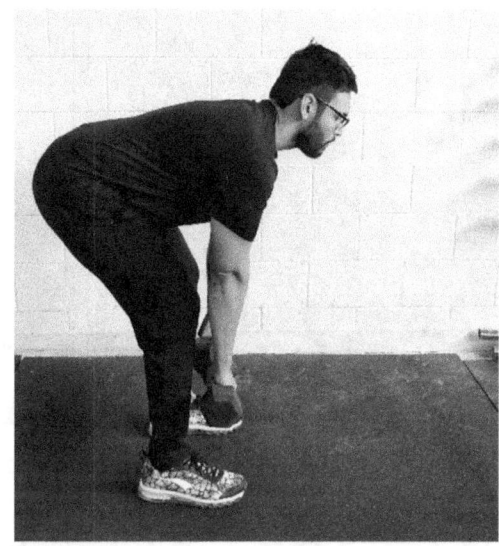

DB Deadlifts 1-2

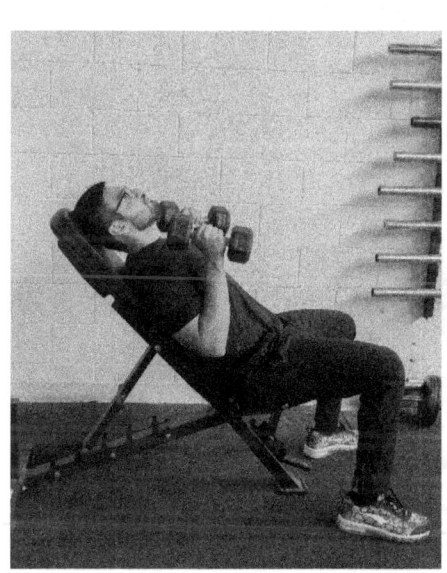 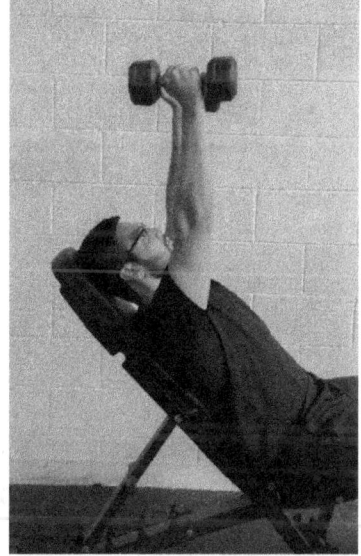

Incline Dumbbell Hammer Press 1-2

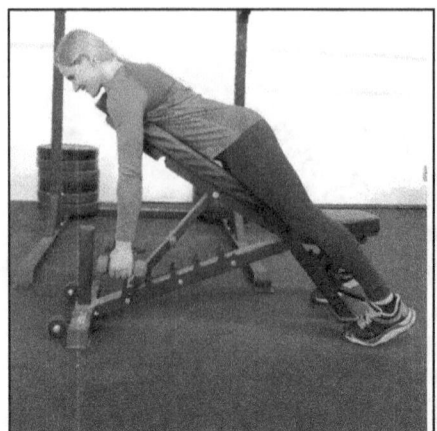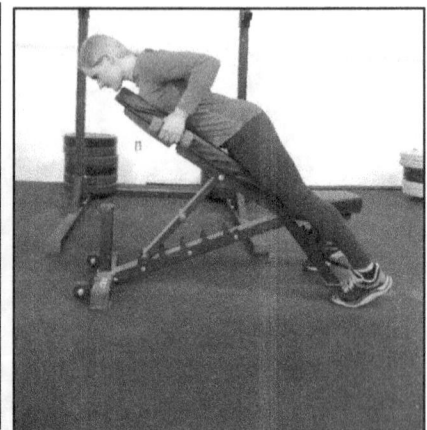

Incline DB Row 1-2

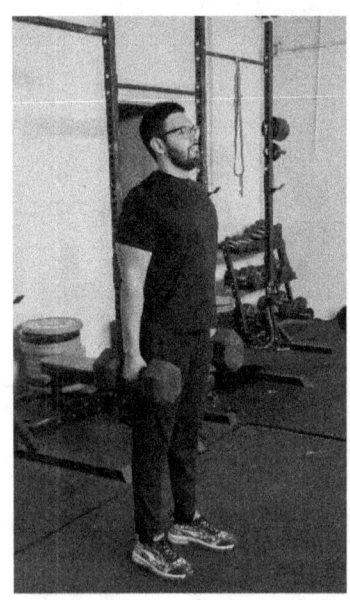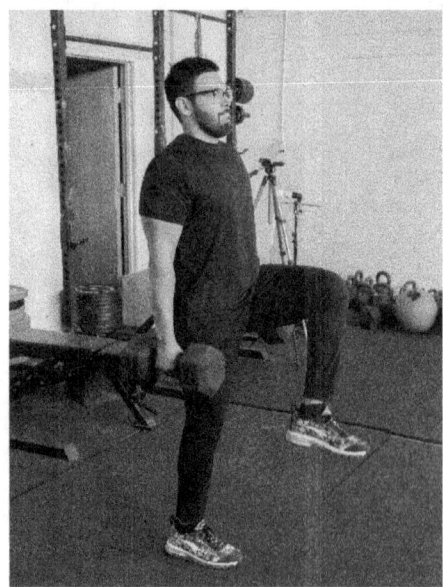

Marching Dumbbell Carry Start

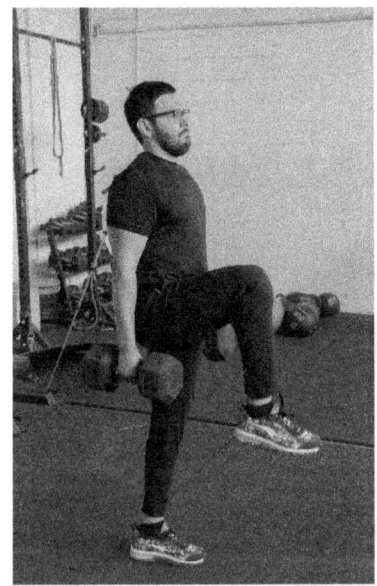
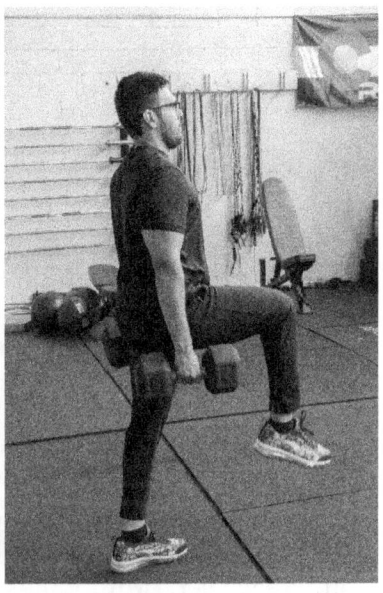
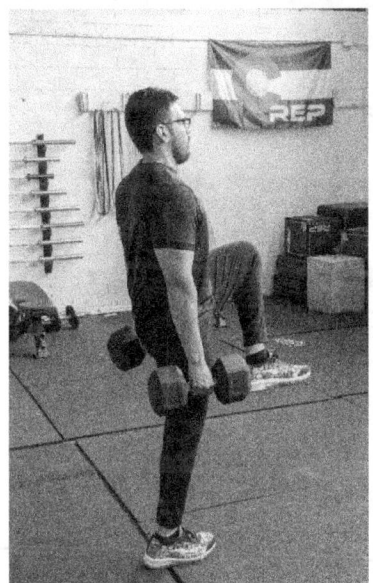

Marching Dumbbell Loaded Carry (Neutral Grip) 1-5

~Week 2~

Dynamic Warm-up:

1. Thread the needle w/ Foam Roller @10-15 repetitions each side.

2. Inch Worms @10-15 repetitions each side.

3. Seated Wall Slides @10-15 reps each side.

Session:

1. Mini-Band Goblet Squat w/ Goblet Setup @15-20 reps, followed by DB Deadlifts @10-15 reps.

   Please complete 4 total sets. *Rest* no more than ninety seconds after each set. (Mini-bands are placed above the knee only for the goblet squat.)

2. **Incline Dumbbell Hammer Press w/twist** @10-15 repetitions, followed by Incline DB Row @10-15 repetitions.

   Please complete 4 total sets. *Rest* no more than sixty seconds after each set.

3. **Marching Dumbbell Loaded Carry (Supinated Grip)** @30-45 seconds, followed by Mountain Climbers @10 each side. (Modify if necessary; please refer to modified Mountain Climber in the Movement Photo Archive.

   Please complete 4 total sets. *Rest* no more than ninety seconds after each set.

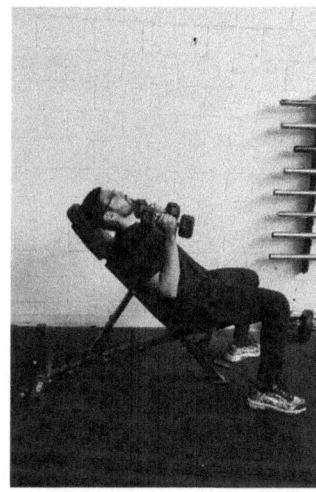 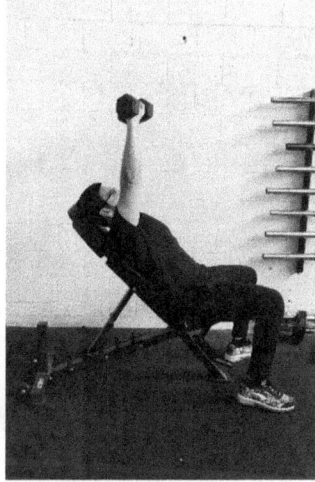

Incline Dumbbell Hammer Press w/twist 1-2

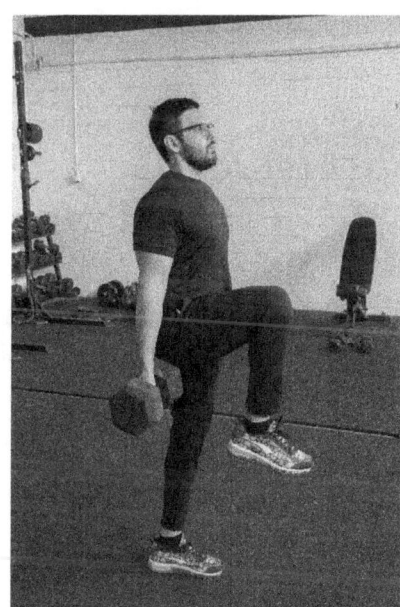 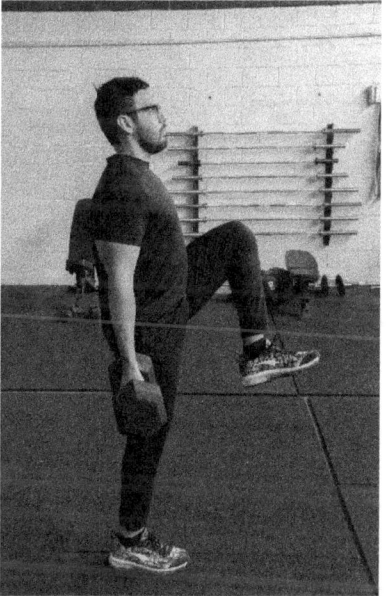

Marching Dumbbell Loaded Carry (Supinated Grip)

~Week 3~

Dynamic Warm-up:

1. Thread the needle w/ Foam Roller @10-15 repetitions each side.

2. Inch Worms @10-15 repetitions each side.

3. Seated Wall Slides @10-15 reps each side.

Session:

1. Mini-band Goblet Squat w/ Goblet Setup @15-20 reps, followed by DB Deadlifts @10-15 reps.

   Please complete 4 total sets. *Rest* no more than ninety seconds after each set. (Mini-bands are placed above the knee only for the goblet squat.)

2. **Incline Dumbbell Hammer Glued Press** @10-15 repetitions, followed by Prone DB Row @10-15 repetitions

   Please complete 4 total sets. *Rest* no more than sixty seconds after each set.

3. Marching Dumbbell Loaded Carry (Neutral Grip) @30-45 seconds, followed by Mountain Climbers @10 each side. (Modify if necessary; please refer to modified Cross Body Mountain Climber in the Movement Photo Archive.

   Please complete 4 total sets. *Rest* no more than ninety seconds after each set.

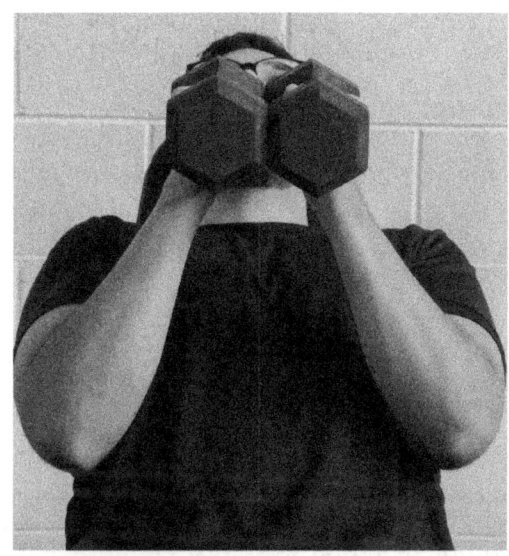

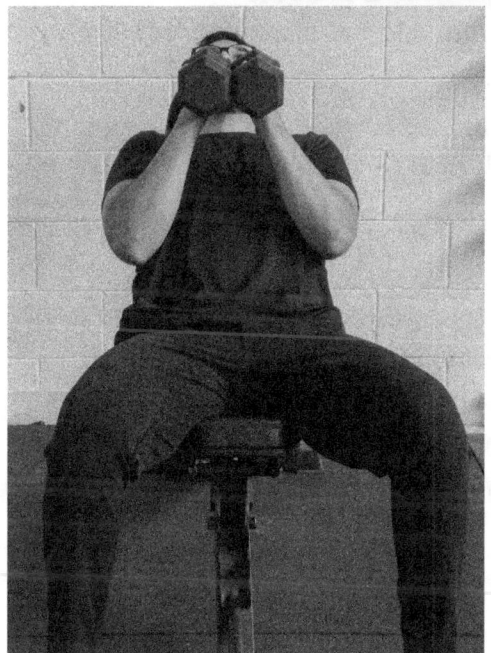
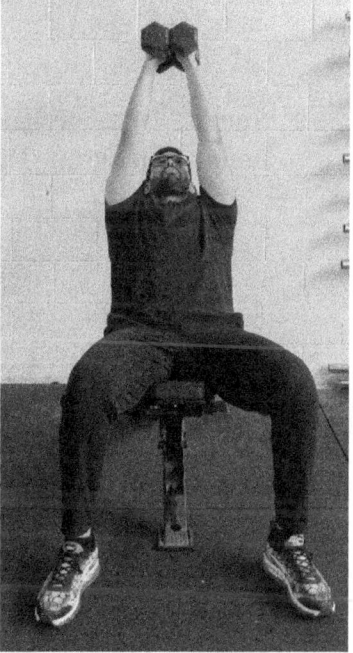

Incline Dumbbell Hammer Glued Press

~Week 4~

Dynamic Warm-up:

1. Thread the needle w/ Foam Roller @10-15 repetitions each side.

2. Inch Worms @10-15 repetitions.

3. Seated Wall Slides @10-15 reps each side.

Session:

1. Mini-band Goblet Squat w/ Goblet Setup @15-20 reps, followed by DB Deadlifts @10-15 reps.

   Please complete 4 total sets. *Rest* no more than ninety seconds after each set. (Mini-bands are placed above the knee only for the goblet squat.)

2. Incline Dumbbell Hammer Glued Press @10-15 repetitions, followed by Prone DB Row @10-15 repetitions

   Please complete 4 total sets. *Rest* no more than sixty seconds after each set.

3. Marching Dumbbell Loaded Carry (Supinated Grip) @30-45 seconds, followed by Mountain Climbers @10 each side. (Modify if necessary; please refer to modified Mountain Climber in the Movement Photo Archive.)

   Please complete 4 total sets. *Rest* no more than ninety seconds after each set.

MONTH #3

WEEKS 1-4

~Week 1~

Dynamic Warm-up:

1. **Rotary Stability** @10 repetitions each side.

2. Inch Worms @15 repetitions each side.

3. **Lizard Lunges** @10 repetitions each side.

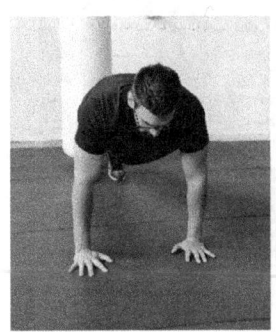 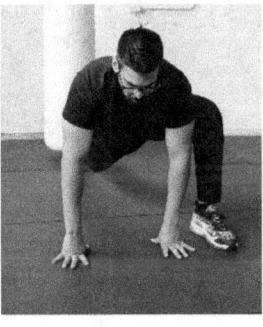 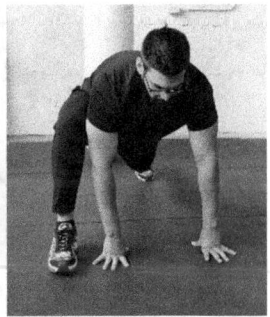

Lizard Lunges 1-3

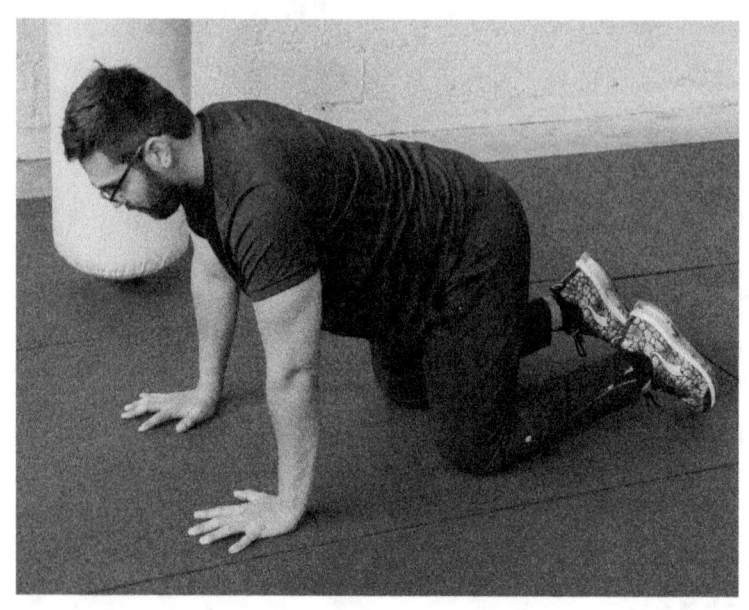

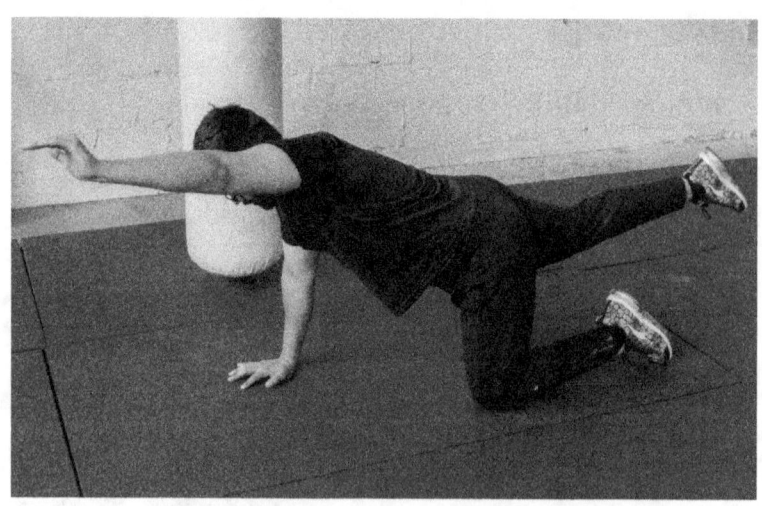

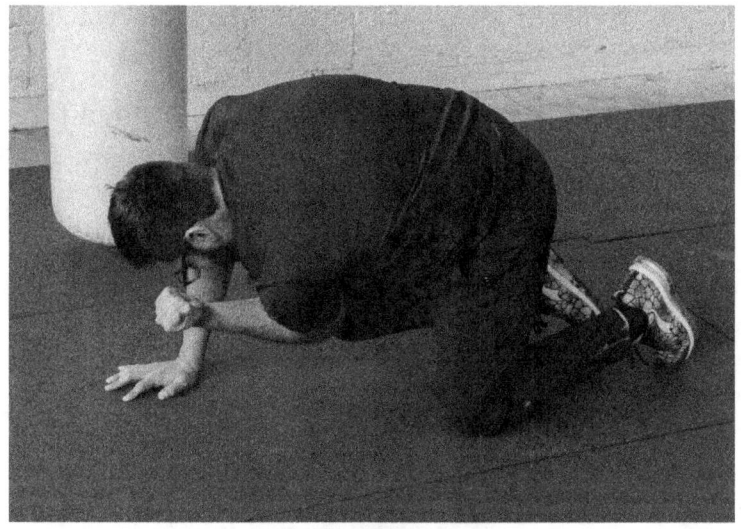

Rotary Stability 1-3

Session:

1. **Double Mini-band Goblet Squat w/ Goblet Setup** @15-20 reps, followed by **Elevated Glute Bridge with mini-band** above the knee only @15-120 reps.

   Please complete 4 total sets. *Rest* no more than ninety seconds after each set. (Mini-bands are placed above the knee and at the ankles for the goblet squat.)

2. Flat Dumbbell Hammer Press @10-15 repetitions, followed by **Bent-over DB Row** w/hammer grip @10-15 repetitions.

   Please complete 4 total sets. *Rest* no more than sixty seconds after each set.

3. **Standing Med Ball Slams** @30-45 seconds.

Please complete 4 total sets. *Rest* no more than ninety seconds after each set.

Take reps given in the session instructions and split them in half then distribute to both sides equally. E.g., If you are doing 14 reps, perform 7 on each side.

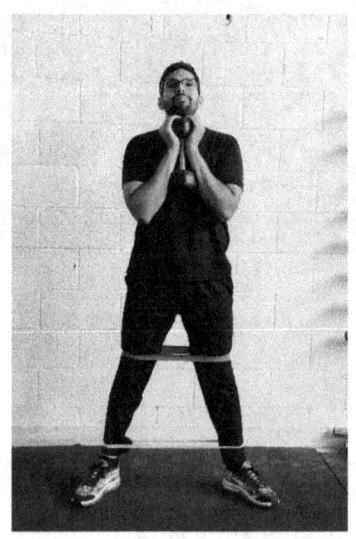

Double Mini-band Goblet Squat w/ Goblet Setup

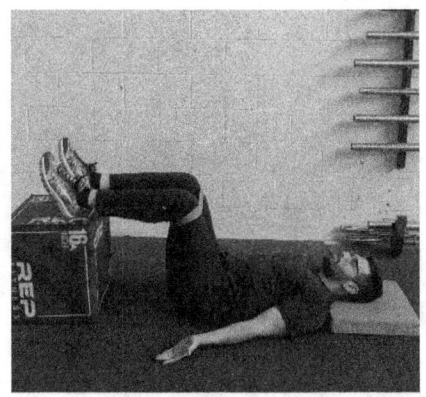 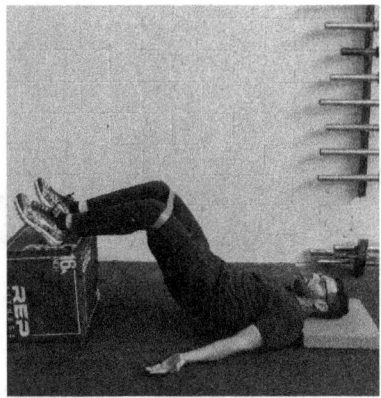

Elevated Glute Bridge with Mini-band above the knee

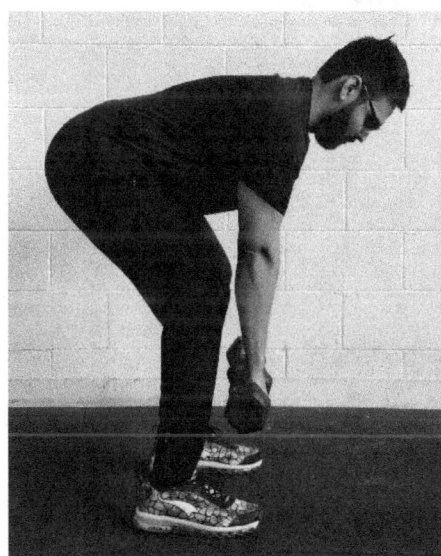 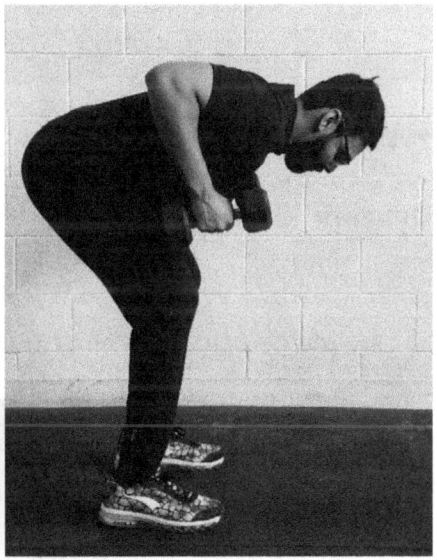

Bent-over DB Row w/twist 1-2

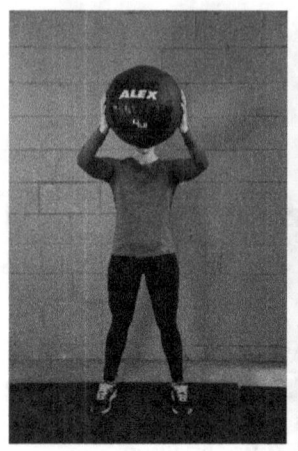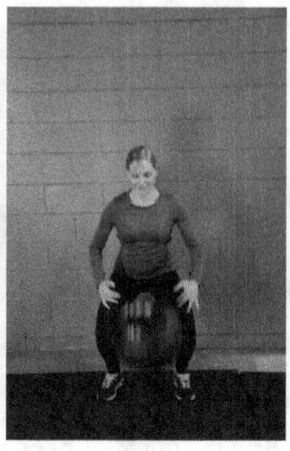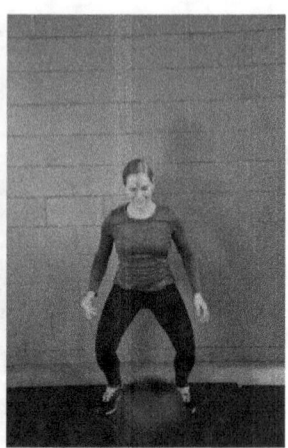

Standing Med Ball Slams 1-3

~Week 2~

Dynamic Warm-up:

1. Rotary Stability @10 repetitions each side.

2. Inch Worms @15 repetitions each side.

3. Lizard Lunges @10 repetitions each side.

Session:

1. Double Mini-band Goblet Squat w/ Goblet Setup @15-20 reps, followed by Elevated Glute Bridge with mini-band @15-120 reps.

   Please complete 4 total sets. *Rest* no more than ninety seconds after each set. (Mini-bands are placed above the knee and at the ankles for the goblet squat.)

2. **Flat Dumbbell Hammer Press** w/twist @10-15 repetitions, followed by Bent-over DB Row w/twist @10-15 repetitions.

   Please complete 4 total sets. *Rest* no more than sixty seconds after each set.

3. Full Kneeling Med Ball Slams @30-45 seconds.

   Please complete 4 total sets. *Rest* no more than ninety seconds after each set.

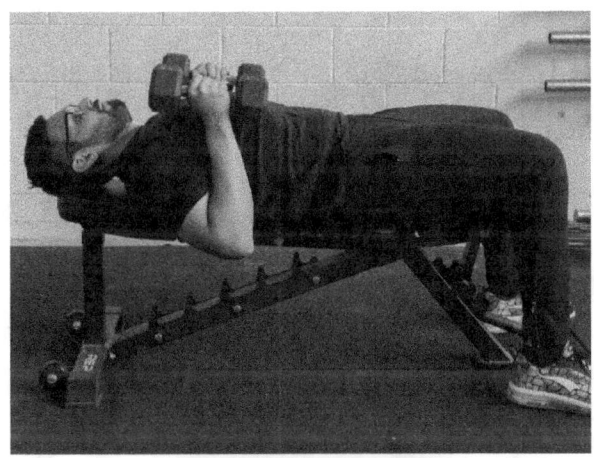

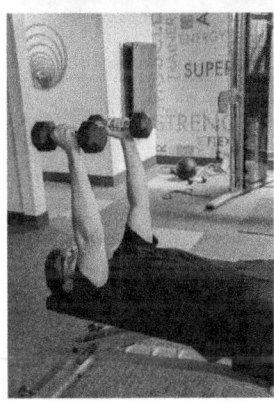

Flat Dumbbell Hammer Press 1-2

~Week 3~

Dynamic Warm-up:

1. Rotary Stability @10 repetitions each side.

2. Inch Worms @15 repetitions each side.

3. Lizard Lunges @10 repetitions each side.

Session:

1. Double Mini-band Goblet Squat w/ Goblet Setup @15-20 reps, followed by Elevated Glute Bridge with mini-band @15-120 reps.

   Please complete 4 total sets. *Rest* no more than ninety seconds after each set. (Mini-bands are placed above the knee and at the ankles for the goblet squat.)

2. Flat Dumbbell Hammer Press @10-15 repetitions, followed by Bent-over DB Row w/hammer grip @10-15 repetitions.

   Please complete 4 total sets. *Rest* no more than sixty seconds after each set.

3. Standing Med Ball Slams @30-45 seconds.

   Please complete 4 total sets. *Rest* no more than ninety seconds after each set.

~Week 4~

Dynamic Warm-up:

1. Rotary Stability @10 repetitions each side.

2. Inch Worms @15 repetitions each side.

3. Lizard Lunges @10 repetitions each side.

Session:

1. Double Mini-band Goblet Squat w/ Goblet Setup @15-20 reps, followed by Elevated Glute Bridge with mini-band @15-120 reps.
   Please complete 4 total sets. *Rest* no more than ninety seconds after each set. (Mini-bands are placed above the knee and at the ankles for the goblet squat.)

2. **Flat Dumbbell Hammer Press w/twist** @10-15 repetitions, followed by **Bent-over DB Row w/twist** @10-15 repetitions.

   Please complete 4 total sets. *Rest* no more than sixty seconds after each set.

3. **Full Kneeling Med Ball Slams** @30-45 seconds.

   Please complete 4 total sets. *Rest* no more than ninety seconds after each set.

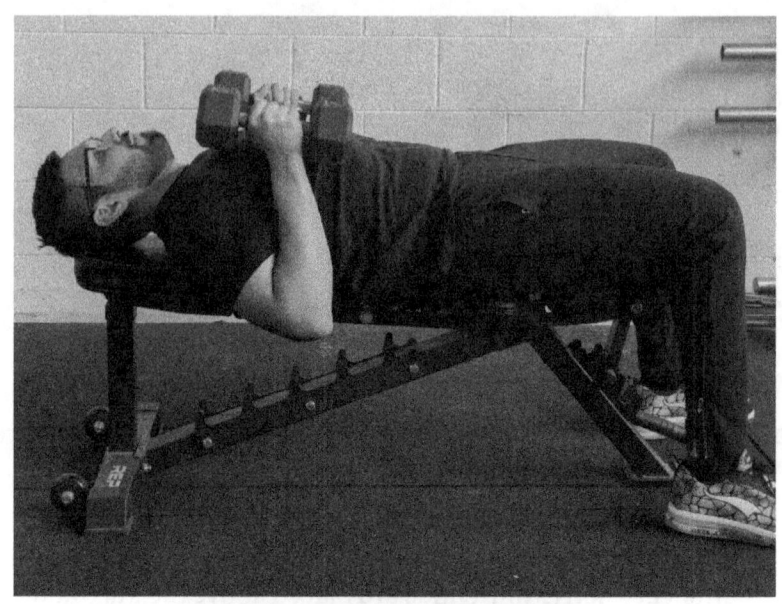

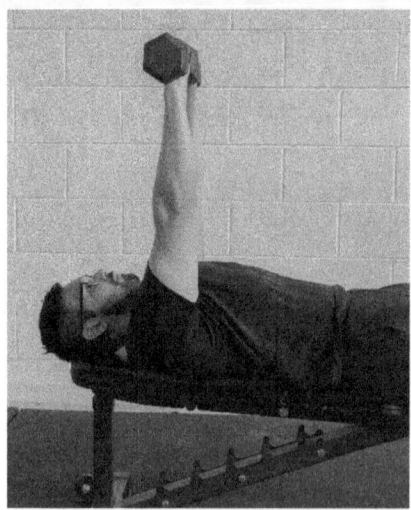

Flat Dumbbell Hammer Press w/twist 1-2

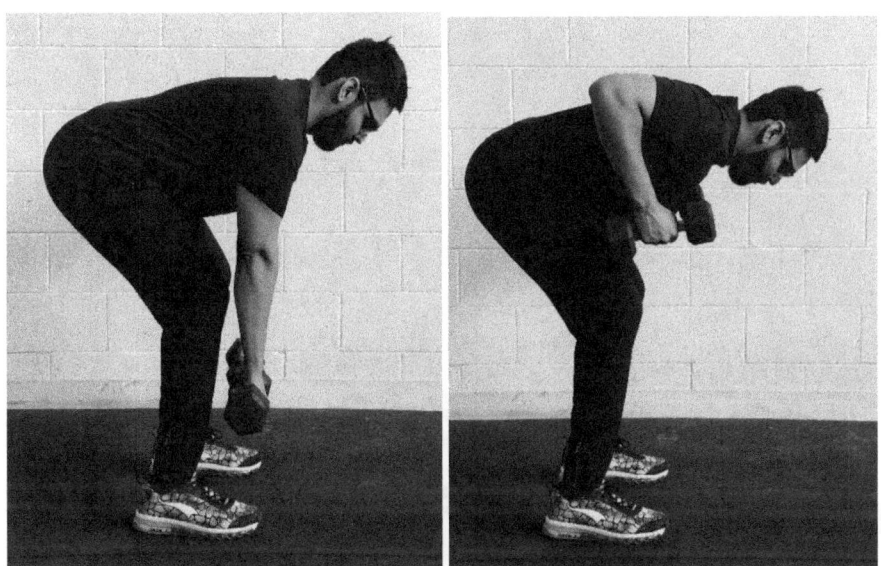

Bent-over DB Row w/twist 1-2

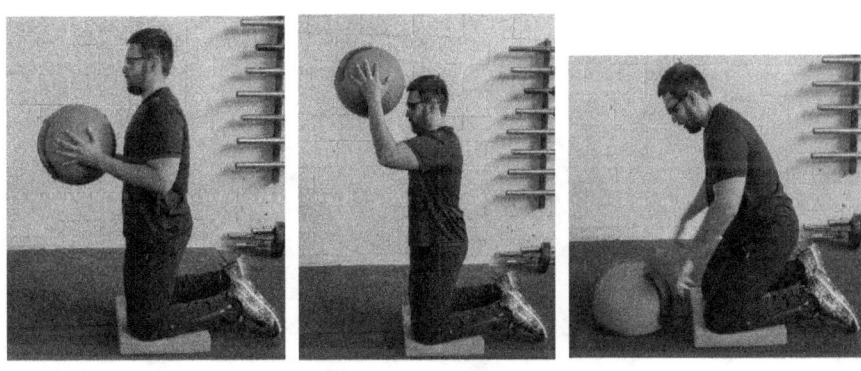

Full Kneeling Med Ball Slams 1-3

WILLIAM RAMON

III.

Second Trimester Fitness Program

WILLIAM RAMON

CHAPTER 3

MONTHS 4-6

NOW THAT WE ARE much stronger, more consistent, and acclimated to a program, it's time to switch gears.

For the first trimester, we focused on developing consistency through discipline, learning the fundamentals, and setting the foundation we need to advance in the program.

For the next three months, we are going to focus on training our muscular imbalances. Muscular imbalances are quite common and exist for a number of reasons, one of which is our lifestyle.

Excess sitting, standing, and frequent inactivity all contribute to imbalances in our muscular strength and flexibility.

To reduce the severity of any current asymmetries, we will be introducing single-extremity movements. When muscular balance is improved, we will not only be stronger and move better in space, but we will feel better overall as well.

Recommended Tools for Maximal Results (Months 4-6)

* Mini-bands
* Foam Roller
* Balance Pad

MONTH #4

WEEKS 1-4

~Week #1~

Dynamic Warm-up:

1. **T-Spine w/ Side Lunge Setup** @10-15 repetitions each side.

2. 5 inchworms plus 5 **World's Greatest Stretch** on each side.

3. **Roller on the Wall** @10-15 repetitions

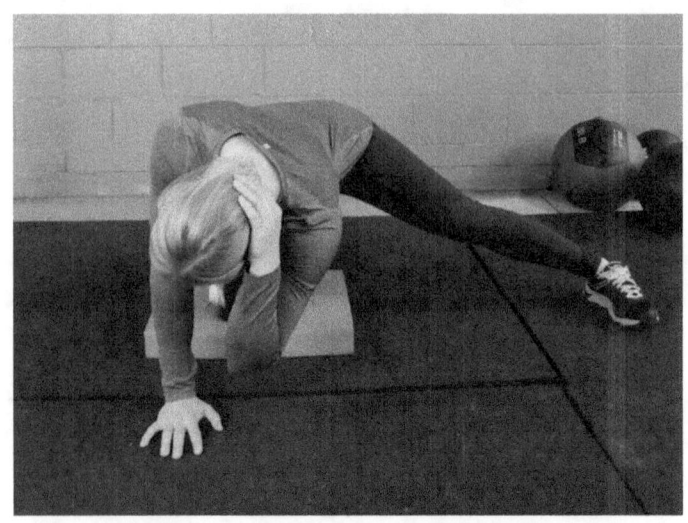

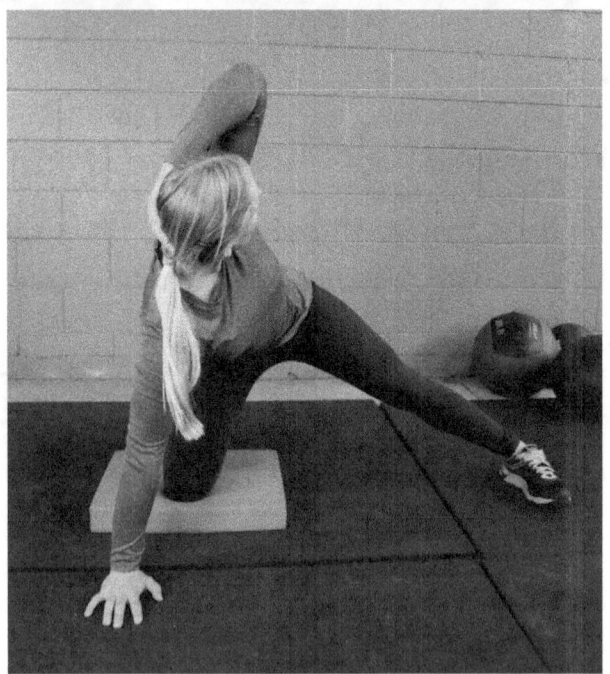

T-Spine w/ Side Lunge Setup 1-2

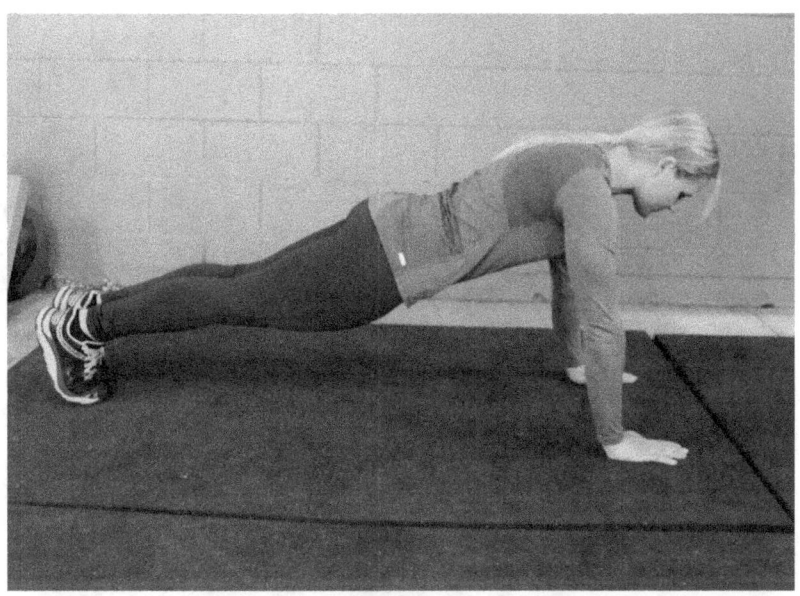

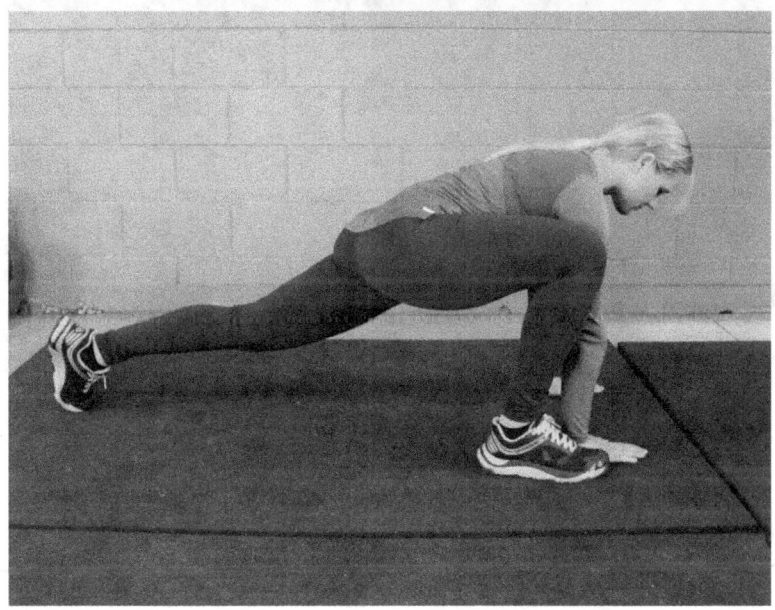

World's Greatest Stretch start

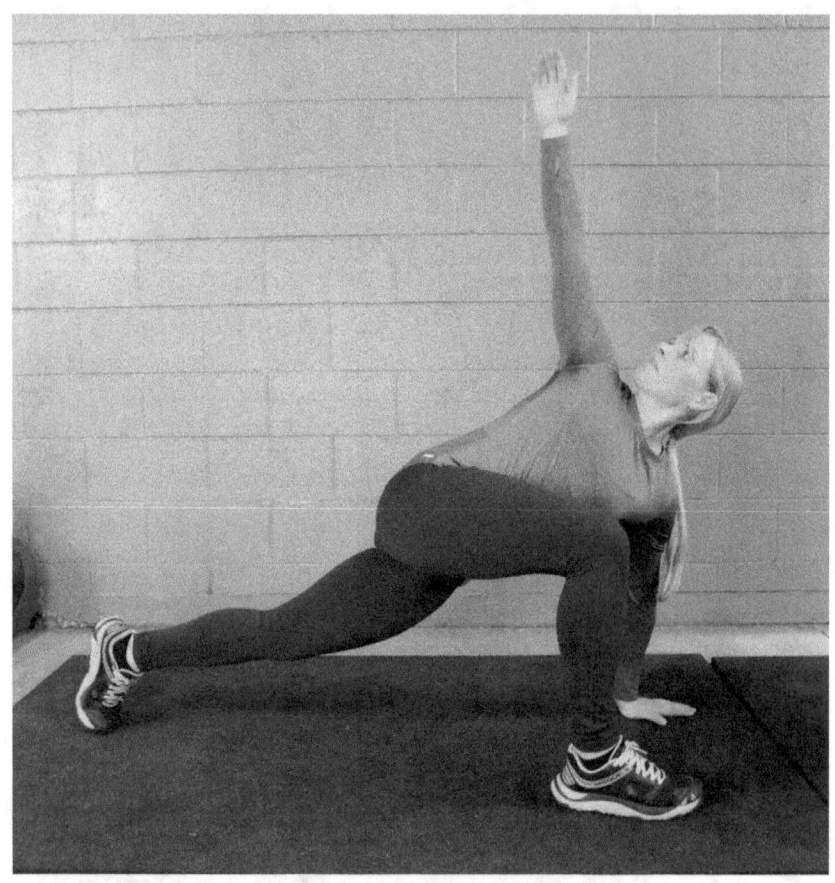

World's Greatest Stretch 1-3

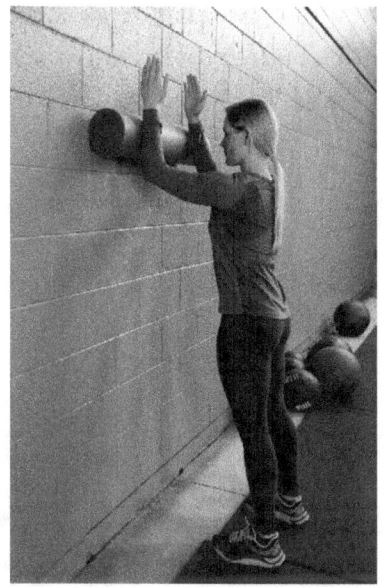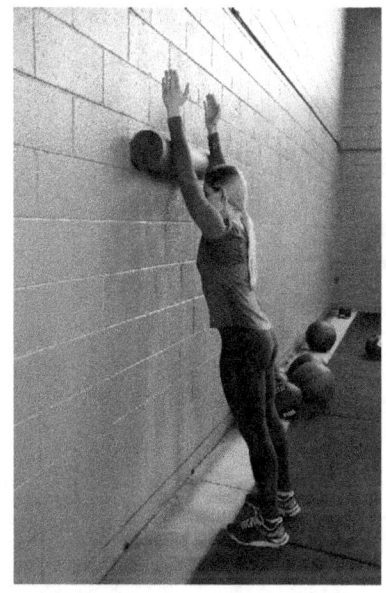

Roller on the Wall

Session:

1. **Single-Leg Step-Up** @15-20 reps, followed by **Single-Leg Glute Bridge** @15-20 reps.

    Please complete 4 total sets. *Rest* no more than ninety seconds after each set.

2. **Single-Arm DB or KB Press on floor** @15-20 repetitions, followed by Standing Single-arm DB Row (Neutral Grip) @15-20 repetitions.

    Please complete 4 total sets. *Rest* no more than sixty seconds after each set.

3. **Single-arm Suitcase Carry (Neutral Grip)** @30-45 seconds, followed by **Calf Raises w/feet pointing straight forward** @25 repetitions.

Please complete 4 total sets. *Rest* no more than sixty seconds after each set.

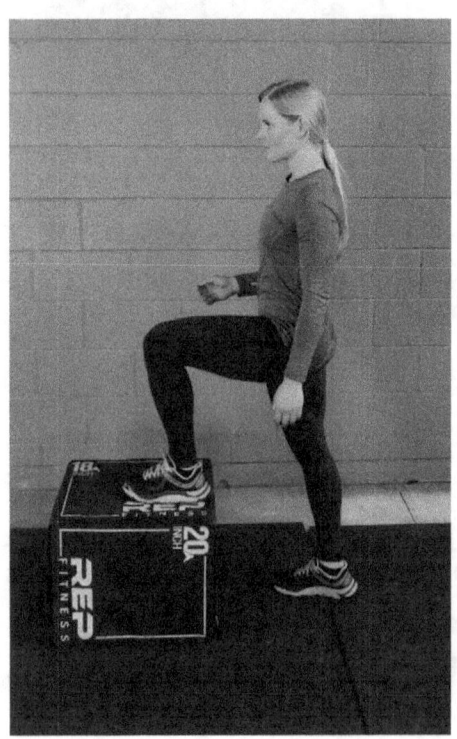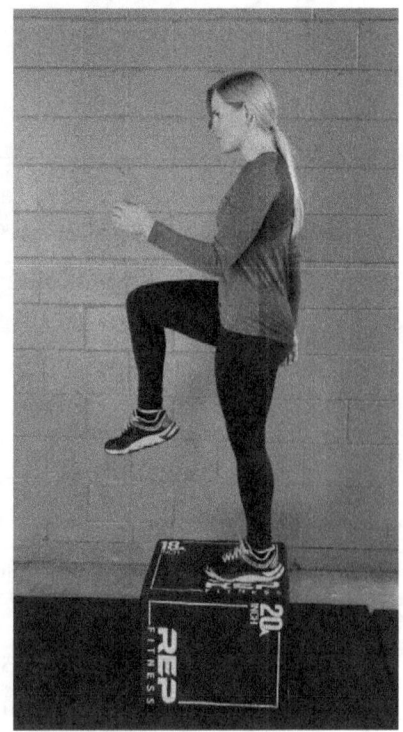

Single-Leg Step-up Start

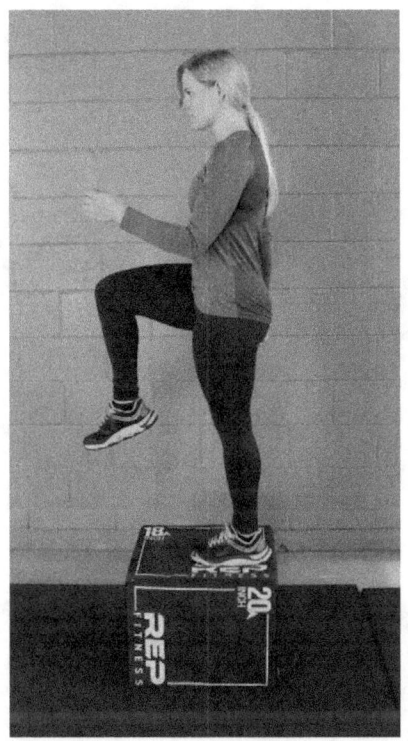

Single-Leg Step-Up 1-3

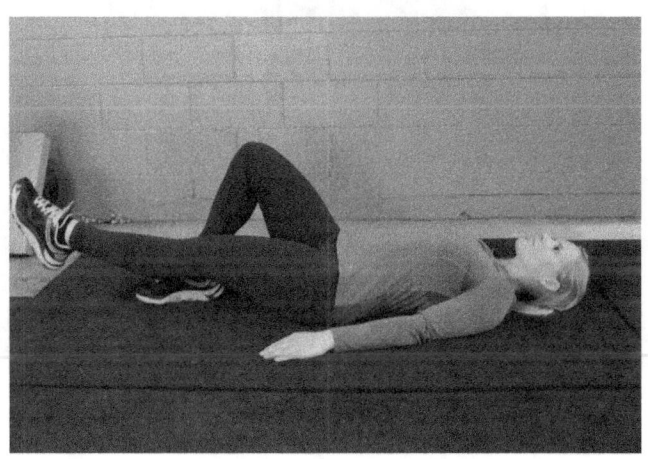

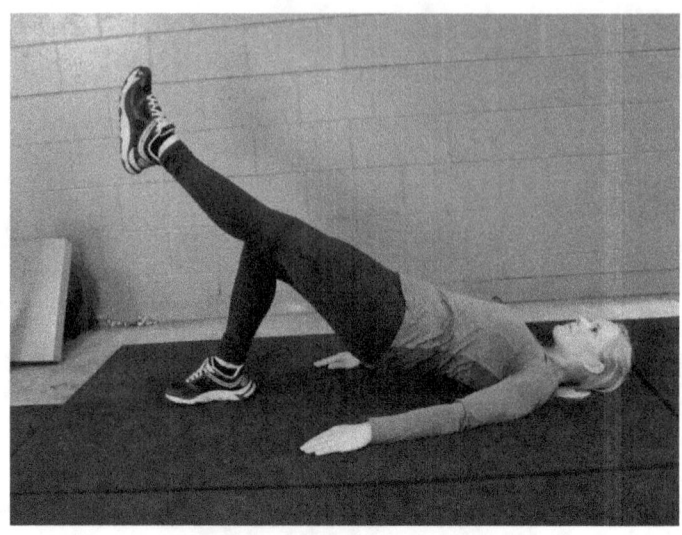

Single-Leg Glute Bridge 1-2

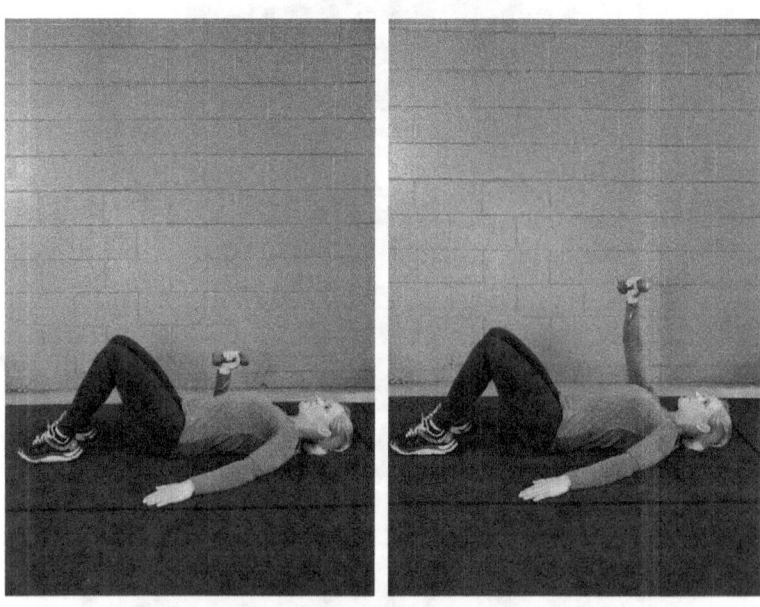

Single-Arm DB or KB Press on floor 1-2

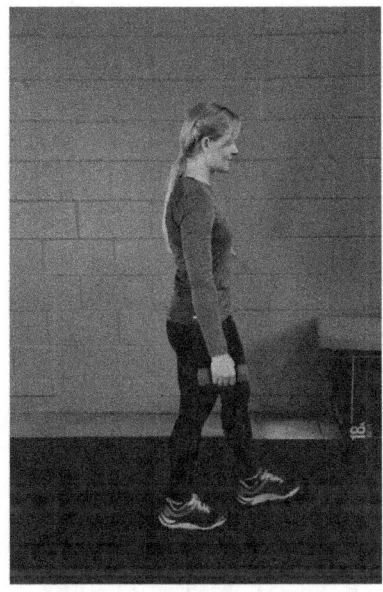 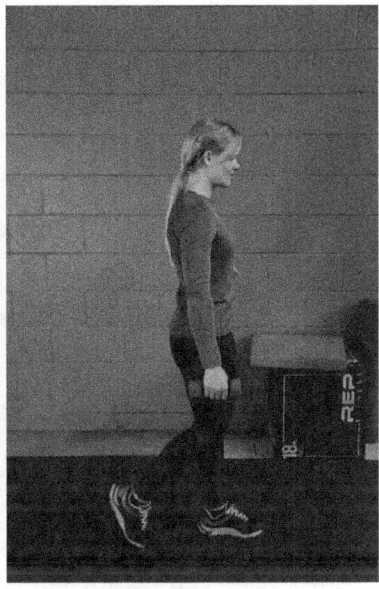

Single-arm Suitcase Carry (Neutral Grip)

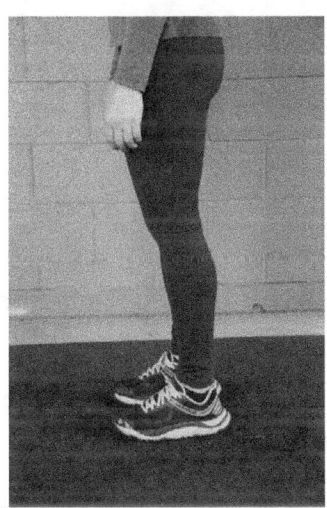 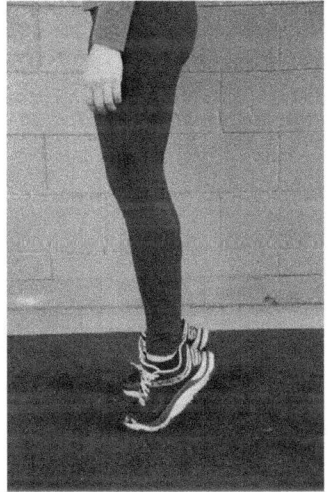

Calf Raises Feet Pointing Forward 1-2

~Week #2~

Dynamic Warm-up:

1. T-Spine w/ Side Lunge Setup @10-15 repetitions each side.

2. 5 inchworms plus 5 World's Greatest on each side.

3. Roller on the Wall @10-15 repetitions.

Session:

1. **Single-leg Lateral 3 Point Step** @15-20 reps each leg, followed by Single-leg Glute Bridge w/ mini-band above the knee @15-20 reps each leg.

   Please complete 4 total sets. *Rest* no more than ninety seconds after each set. (Mini-bands are placed at the ankle only for the three-point step.)

2. Single-arm DB or KB Press on floor @15-20 repetitions, followed by Standing Single-arm DB Row w/twist (pronated to neutral grip) @15-20 repetitions.

   Please complete 4 total sets. *Rest* no more than sixty seconds after each set.

3. Single-arm **Suitcase Carry (Supinated Grip)** @30-45 seconds, followed by **Calf Raises w/feet pointing outwards** @25 repetitions.

   Please complete 4 total sets. *Rest* no more than sixty seconds after each set.

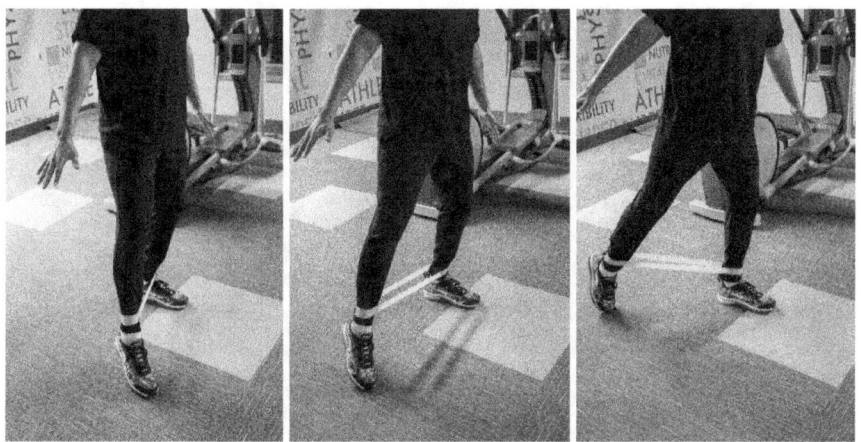

Single-leg Lateral 3-Point Steps, 1-3

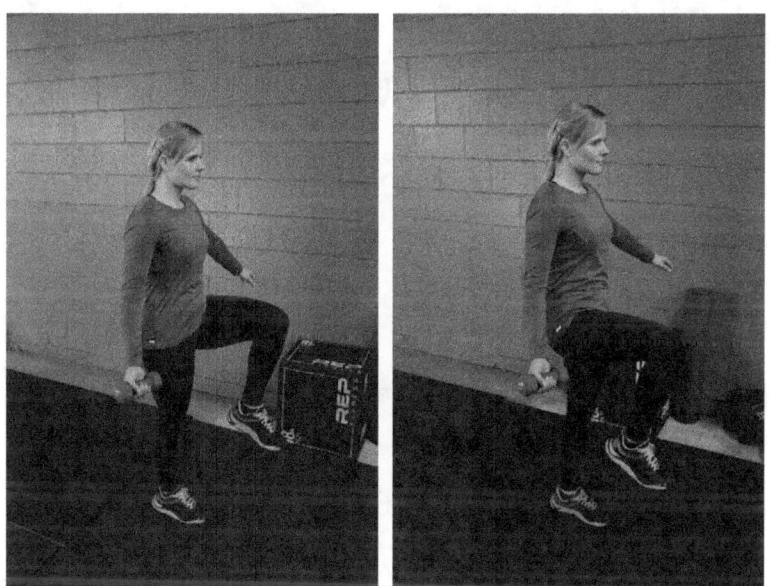

Single-arm Marching Suitcase Carry (Supinated Grip) 1-2

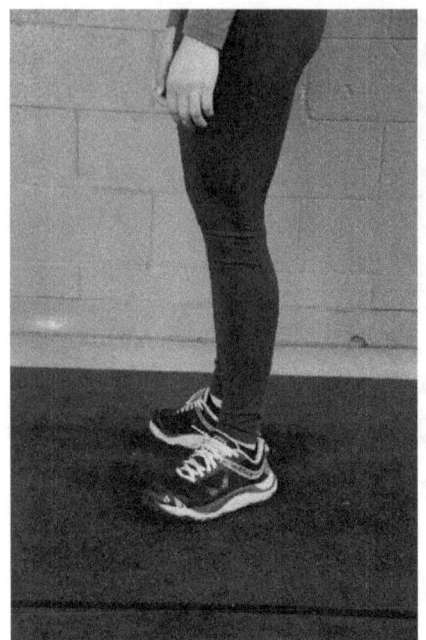 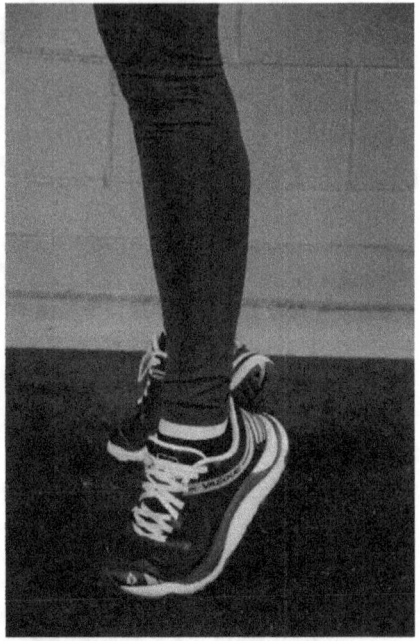

Calf Raises Feet Pointing Outward

~Week #3~

Dynamic Warm-up:

1. T-Spine w/ Side Lunge Setup @10-15 repetitions each side.

2. 5 inchworms plus 5 World's Greatest on each side.

3. Roller on the Wall @10-15 repetitions

Session:

1. Single-leg Step Up @15-20 reps, followed by Single-leg Glute Bridge @15-20 reps.

   Please complete 4 total sets. *Rest* no more than ninety seconds after each set.

2. Single-arm DB or KB Press on floor @15-20 repetitions, followed by Standing Single-arm DB Row (Neutral Grip) @15-20 repetitions.

   Please complete 4 total sets. *Rest* no more than sixty seconds after each set.

3. Single-arm Suitcase Carry (Neutral Grip) @30-45 seconds, followed by Calf Raises w/feet pointing straight forward @25 repetitions.

   Please complete 4 total sets. *Rest* no more than sixty seconds after each set.

~Week #4~

Dynamic Warm-up:

1. T-Spine w/ Side Lunge Setup @10-15 repetitions each side.
2. 5 inchworms plus 5 World's Greatest on each side.
3. Roller on the Wall @10-15 repetitions

Session:

1. Single-leg Lateral 3-Point Step @15-20 reps each leg, followed by **Single-leg Glute Bridge w/ mini-band above the knee** @15-20 reps each leg.

   Please complete 4 total sets. *Rest* no more than ninety seconds after each set. (Mini-bands are placed at the ankle only for the 3-point step.)

2. Single-arm DB or KB Press on floor @15-20 repetitions, followed by Standing Single-arm DB Row w/twist (pronated to neutral grip) @15-20 repetitions.

   Please complete 4 total sets. *Rest* no more than sixty seconds after each set.

3. Single-arm Suitcase Carry (Supinated Grip) @30-45 seconds, followed by Calf Raises w/feet pointing outwards @25 repetitions.

   Please complete 4 total sets. *Rest* no more than sixty seconds after each set.

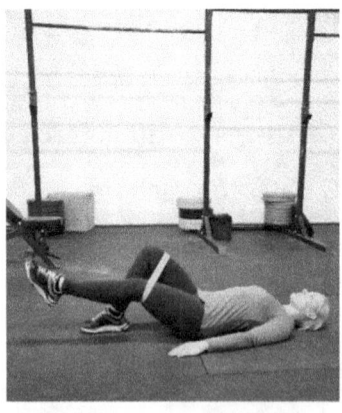 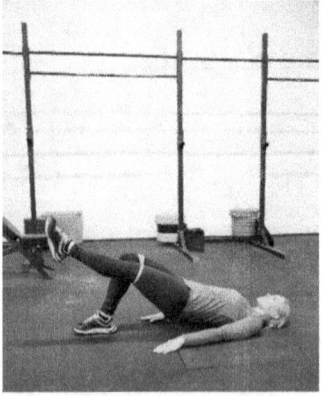

Single-leg Glute Bridge w/ mini-band above the knee

MONTH #5

WEEKS 1-4

~Week #1~

Dynamic Warm-up:

1. T-Spine w/ Side Lunge Setup @10-15 repetitions each side.
2. 5 inchworms plus 5 World's Greatest on each side.
3. **Mini-Band Wall Crawl** @10-15 repetitions.

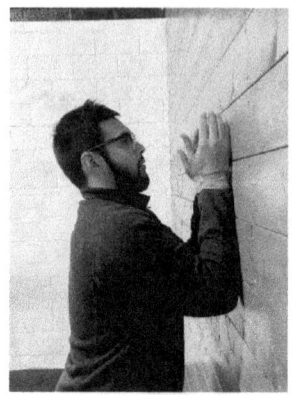 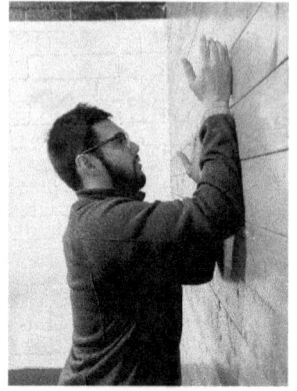 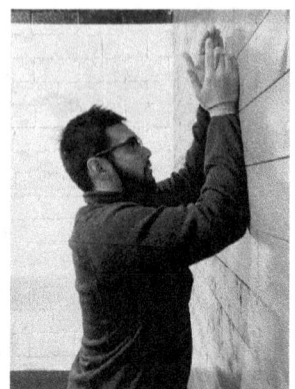

Mini-Band Wall Crawl 1-3
Make sure to fully extend through the tips of your fingers before marching back down slowly

Keep elbows on the wall.

Session:

1. **Mini-band Side Steps** @15-20 reps, followed by **Staggered Stance DB deadlift** @15-20 reps each side.

   Please complete 4 total sets. *Rest* no more than ninety seconds after each set.

2. **Single-arm DB or KB Press on Incline** @20-25 repetitions, followed by Single-leg, Single-arm, **DB Row on bench** (Neutral Grip) @20-25 repetitions.

   Please complete 4 total sets. *Rest* no more than sixty seconds after each set.

3. **Single-arm Marching Suitcase Carry (Neutral Grip)** @30-45 seconds, followed by **Seated Calf Raises** w/feet pointing straight forward @25 repetitions.

FIT & EXPECTING

Add a dumbbell on your lap for resistance. Please complete 4 total sets. *Rest* no more than sixty seconds after each set.

Take reps given in the session instructions and split them in half then distribute to both sides equally. E.g., If you are doing 14 reps, perform 7 on each side.

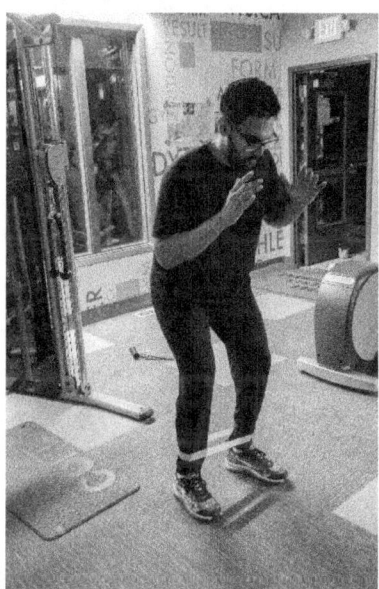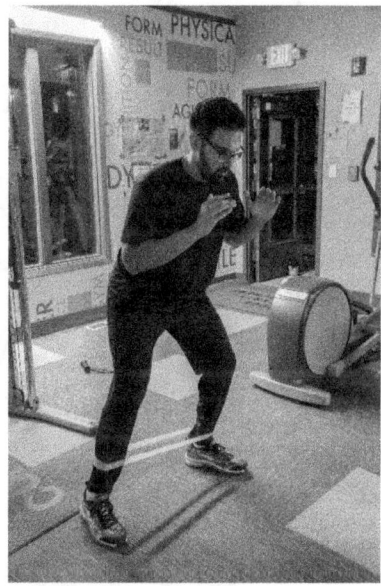

Mini-band Side Steps 1-2

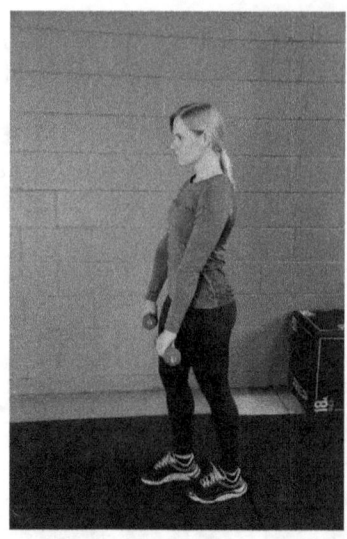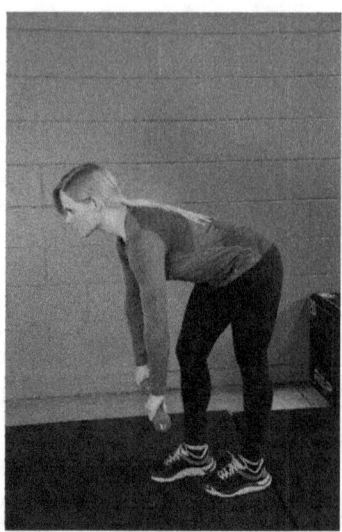

Staggered Stance DB deadlift 1-2

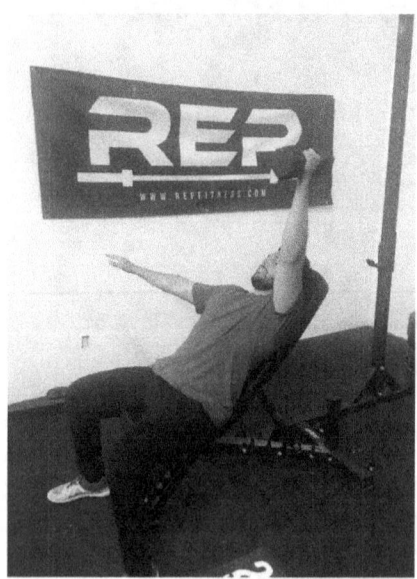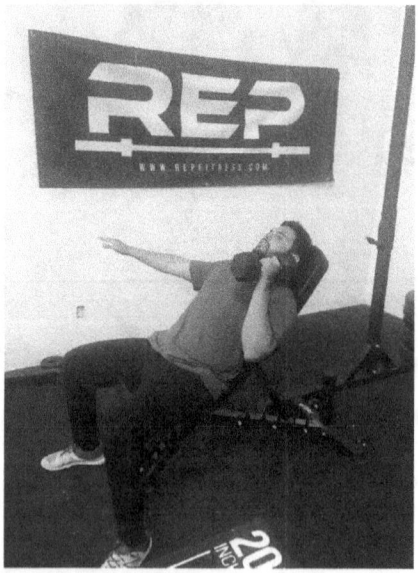

Single-arm DB or KB Press on Incline

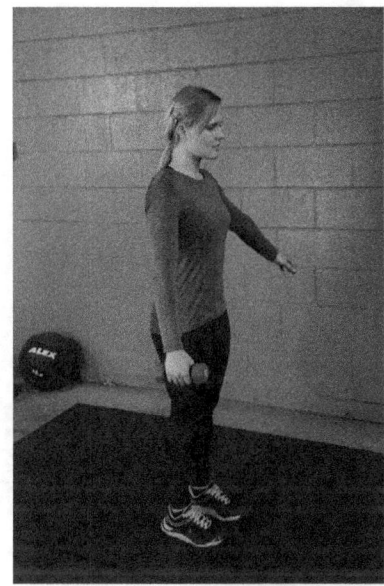
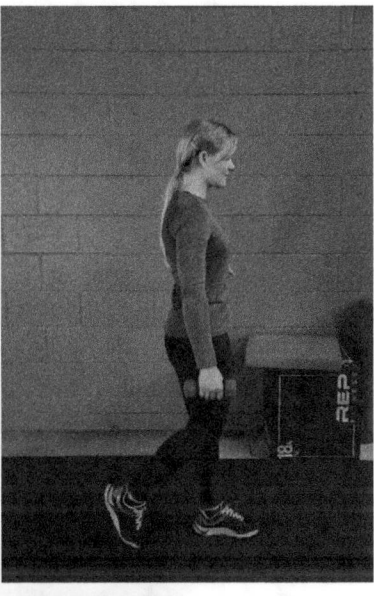
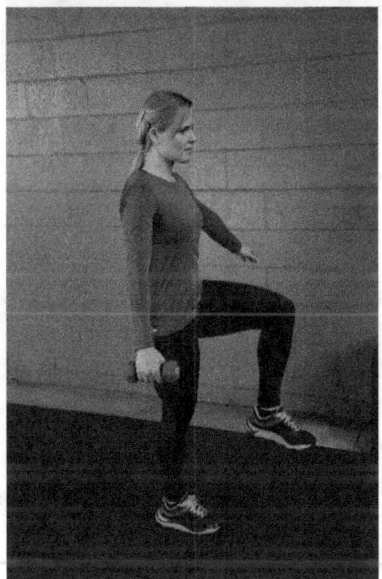

Single-arm Marching Suitcase Carry (Neutral Grip) 1-3

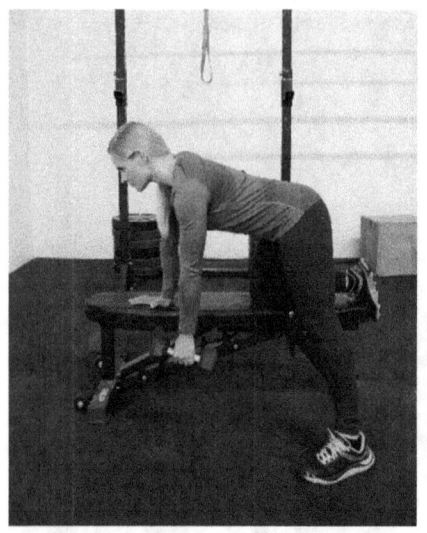 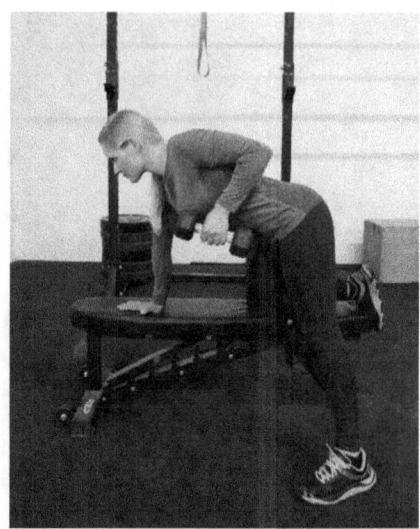

DB Row on Flat Bench

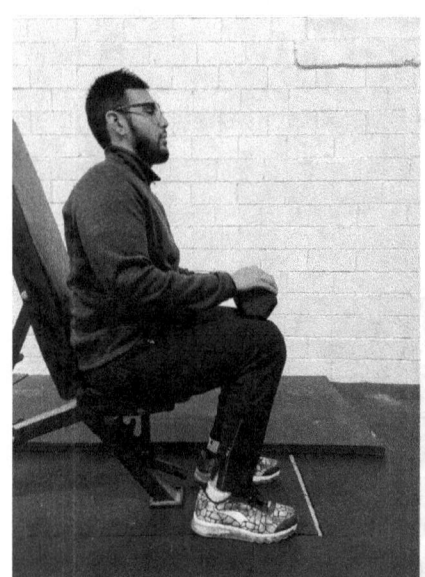 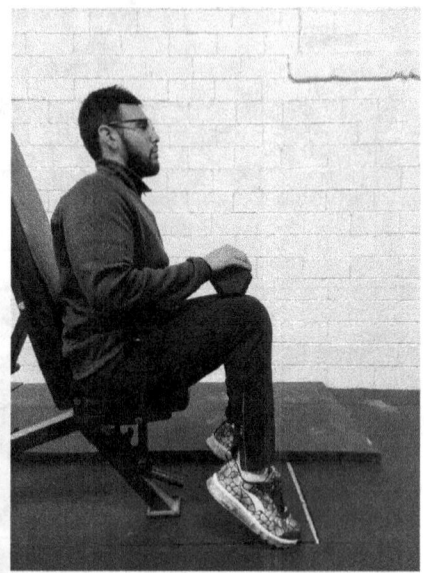

Seated Calf Raises 1-2
Notice how I am off my heels and on my toes in Pic 2.

~Week #2~

Dynamic Warm-up:

1. T-Spine w/ Side Lunge Setup @10-15 repetitions each side.

2. 5 inchworms plus 5 World's Greatest on each side.

3. Mini-band crawl @10-15 repetitions

Session:

1. Mini-band Side Steps @15 reps each side, followed by Staggered Stance DB deadlift @20-25 reps each side.

   Please complete 4 total sets. *Rest* no more than ninety seconds after each set.

2. Single-arm DB or KB Press on Incline @20-25 repetitions, followed by Single-leg, Single-arm, DB Row on bench (Neutral Grip) @20-25 repetitions.

   Please complete 4 total sets. *Rest* no more than sixty seconds after each set.

3. Single-arm Marching Suitcase Carry (Supinated Grip) @30-45 seconds, followed by Seated Calf Raises w/feet pointing straight forward @25 repetitions. Add a dumbbell on your lap for resistance.

   Please complete 4 total sets. *Rest* no more than sixty seconds after each set.

~Week #3~

Dynamic Warm-up:

1. T-Spine w/ Side Lunge Setup @10-15 repetitions each side.

2. 5 inchworms plus 5 World's Greatest on each side.

3. Mini-band crawl @10-15 repetitions.

Session:

1. Mini-band Side Steps @20-25 reps, followed by Staggered Stance DB deadlift @20-25 reps each side.

   Please complete 4 total sets. *Rest* no more than ninety seconds after each set.

2. Single-arm DB or KB Press on Incline 20-25 repetitions, followed by Single-leg, Single-arm, DB Row on bench (Neutral Grip) @20-25 repetitions.

   Please complete 4 total sets. *Rest* no more than sixty seconds after each set.

3. Single-arm Marching Suitcase Carry (Neutral Grip) @30-45 seconds, followed by Seated Calf Raises w/feet pointing straight forward @25 repetitions. Add a dumbbell on your lap for resistance.

   Please complete 4 total sets. *Rest* no more than sixty seconds after each set.

~Week #4~

FIT & EXPECTING

Dynamic Warm-up:

1. T-Spine w/ Side Lunge Setup @10-15 repetitions each side.

2. 5 inchworms plus 5 World's Greatest on each side.

3. Mini-band crawl @10-15 repetitions.

Session:

1. Mini-band Side Steps @25-30 reps each side, followed by Staggered Stance DB deadlift @20-25 reps each side.

   Please complete 4 total sets. *Rest* no more than ninety seconds after each set.

2. Single-arm DB or KB Press on Incline @20-25 repetitions, followed by Single-leg, Single-arm, DB Row on bench (Neutral Grip) @20-25 repetitions.

   Please complete 4 total sets. *Rest* no more than sixty seconds after each set.

3. Single-arm Marching Suitcase Carry (Supinated Grip) @30-45 seconds, followed by Seated Calf Raises w/feet pointing straight forward @25 repetitions. Add a dumbbell on your lap for resistance.

   Please complete 4 total sets. *Rest* no more than sixty seconds after each set.

Recommended Tools for Maximal Results (Months 6-9)

* Mini-bands
* Foam Roller
* Balance Pad

MONTH #6

WEEKS 1-4

~Week #1~

Dynamic Warm-up:

1. **T-Spine w/ band** @15 repetitions each side.

2. World's Greatest @15 repetitions each side.

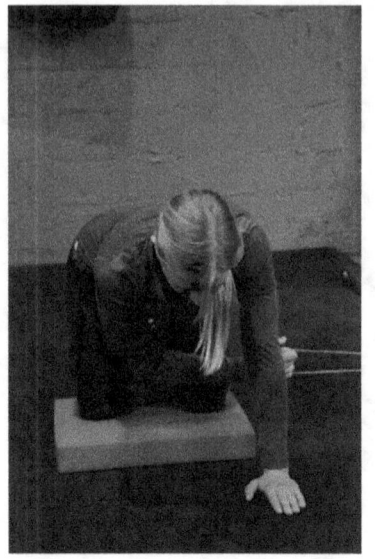 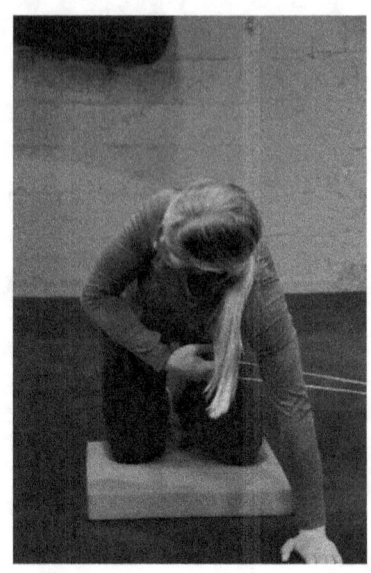

T-Spine w/ band

Session:

1. **Split Stance, Split Squat** @10-15 reps each side, followed by **Reverse Lunge** @10-15 reps each side.

   Please complete 4 total sets. *Rest* no more than ninety seconds after each set.

2. Standing Single-arm Shoulder Press @10-15 repetitions each side.

   Please complete 4 total sets. *Rest* no more than sixty seconds after each set.

3. Single-arm, overhead, Loaded Carry (Neutral Grip) @20-30 seconds, followed by **Single-leg Calf Raise** @10-15 each side. Please complete 4 total sets. *Rest* no more than ninety seconds after each set.

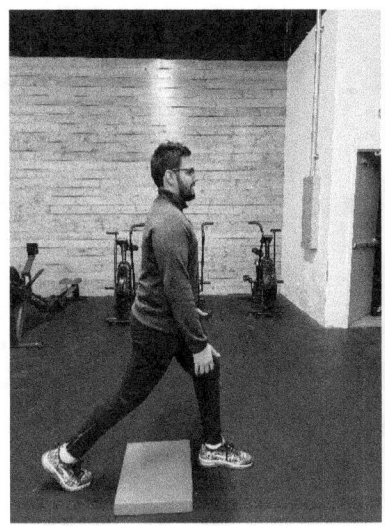
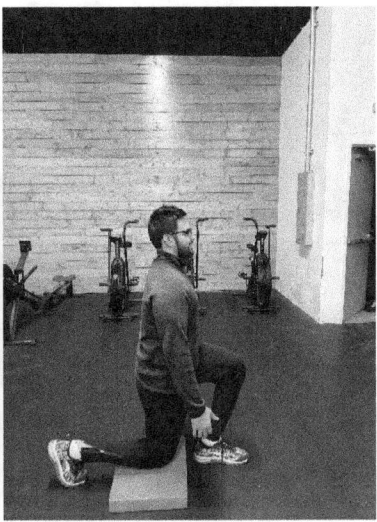

Split Stance, Split Squat

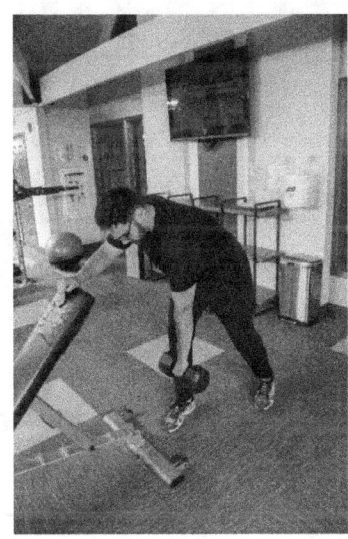
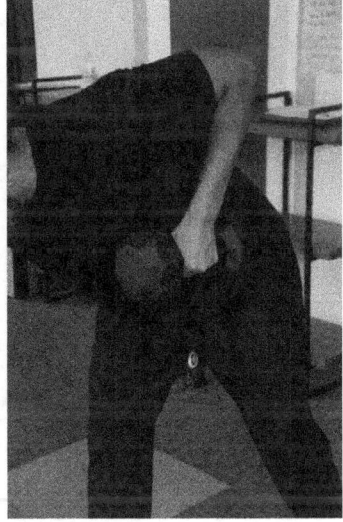

Standing Single Row w/Twist

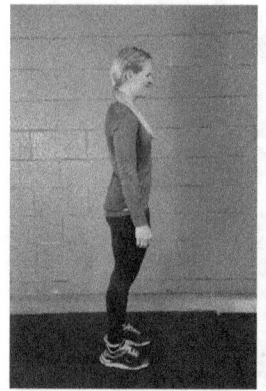 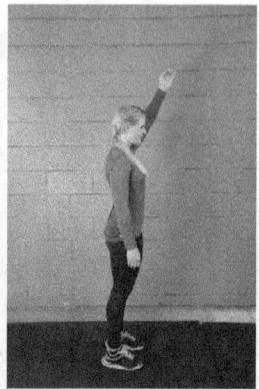 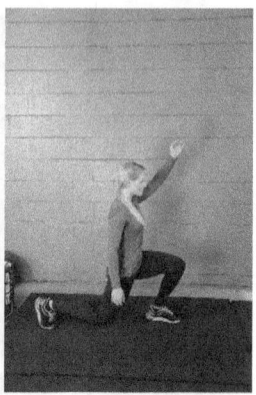

Reverse Lunge

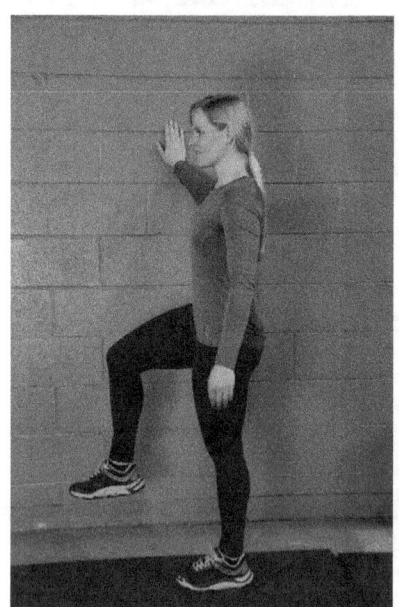 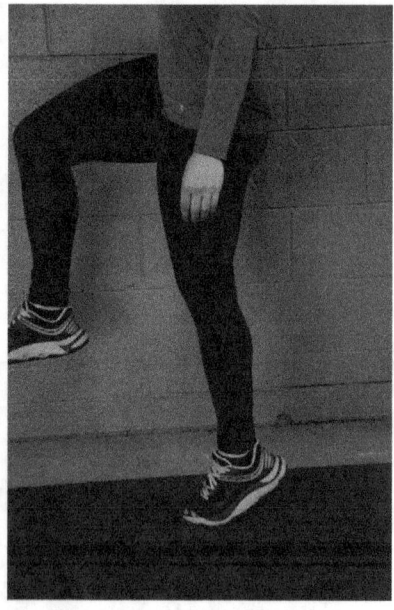

Single-leg Calf Raise

~Week #2~

Dynamic Warm-up:

1. T-Spine w/ band @15 repetitions each side.

2. World's Greatest @10 repetitions each side.

Session:

1. **Bulgarian Split Squat** @10-15 reps each side, followed by Reverse Lunge @10-15 reps each side.

   Please complete 4 total sets. *Rest* no more than ninety seconds after each set.

2. Standing Single-arm Shoulder Press @15-20 repetitions each side.

   Please complete 4 total sets. *Rest* no more than sixty seconds after each set.

3. Single-arm, Overhead, Marching in Place, Loaded Carry (Neutral Grip) @20-30 seconds, followed by Single-leg Calf Raise @10-15 each side.

   Please complete 4 total sets. *Rest* no more than ninety seconds after each set.

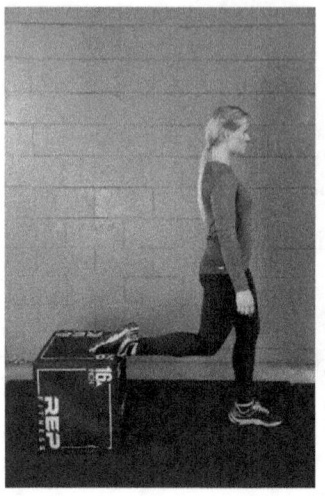 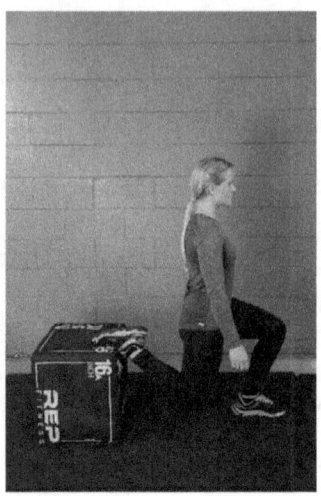

Bulgarian Split Squat 1-2

~Week #3~

Dynamic Warm-up:

1. T-Spine w/ band @15 repetitions each side.

2. World's Greatest @15 repetitions each side.

Session:

1. Split Stance, Split Squat @15-20 reps each side, followed by Reverse Lunge @15-20 reps each side.

   Please complete 4 total sets. *Rest* no more than ninety seconds after each set.

2. **Half-Kneeling Single-arm Shoulder Press** @15-20 repetitions each side.

Please complete 4 total sets. *Rest* no more than sixty seconds after each set.

3. **Single-arm, overhead, Loaded Carry** (Neutral Grip) @30-45 seconds, followed by Single-leg Calf Raise @15-20 each side.

Please complete 4 total sets. *Rest* no more than ninety seconds after each set.

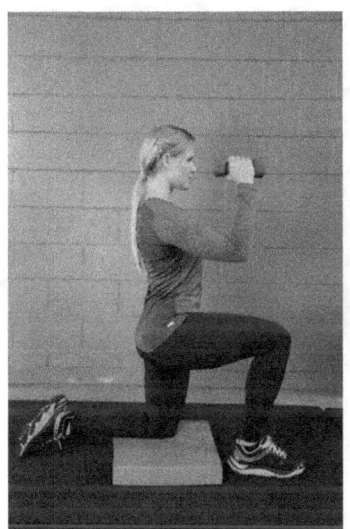 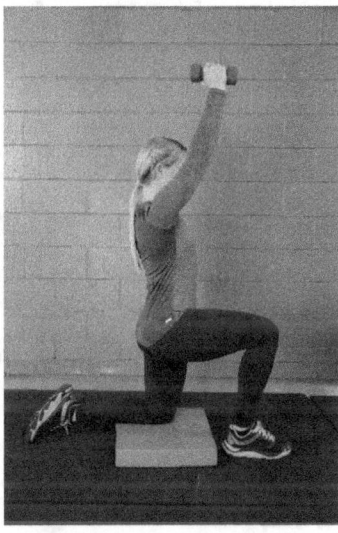

Half-Kneeling Single-arm Shoulder Press 1-2

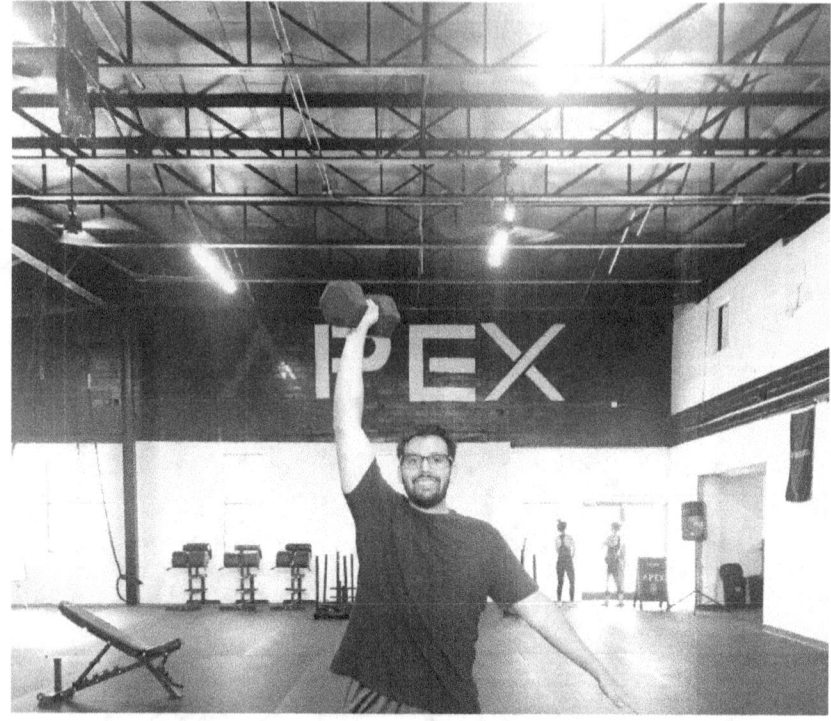

Single-arm, overhead, Loaded Carry

~Week #4~

Dynamic Warm-up:

1. T-Spine w/ band @15 repetitions each side.
2. World's Greatest @15 repetitions each side.

Session:

1. Bulgarian Split Squat @15-20 reps each side, followed by Reverse Lunge @15-20 reps each side.

   Please complete 4 total sets. *Rest* no more than ninety seconds after each set.

2. Half Kneeling Single-arm Shoulder Press @15-20 repetitions each side.

   Please complete 4 total sets. *Rest* no more than sixty seconds after each set.

3. Single-arm, Overhead, Marching in Place, Loaded Carry (Neutral Grip) @20-30 seconds, followed by Single-leg Calf Raise @15-20 each side.

   Please complete 4 total sets. *Rest* no more than ninety seconds after each set.

WILLIAM RAMON

IV.

Third Trimester Fitness Program

WILLIAM RAMON

CHAPTER 4

MONTHS 7-9

FIRST AND FOREMOST, I would like you to take this very moment to celebrate with yourself for reaching this point in the program. It is a job well done!

Now, for the most important part: the final trimester. In this three-month cycle, we will focus more on compound movements. These movements will not only make you stronger, but they will help take your muscle building, calorie burning, and total fat loss to the next level!

MONTH #7

WEEKS 1-4

~Week #1~

Dynamic Warm-up:

1. T-Spine w/ Side Lunge Setup @10-15 repetitions each side.

2. 5 inchworms plus World's Greatest on each side.

3. Roller on the Wall @10-15 repetitions

Session:

1. **Dumbbell Thrusters** @10-15 reps, followed by **Reverse Band Walk** @30-45 seconds.

   Please complete 4 total sets. *Rest* no more than ninety seconds after each set.

2. **Single-arm Split Stance Band or Cable Press** 15-20 repetitions each side, followed by **Modified Pull-up, i.e., inverted row** @15-20 repetitions.

   Please complete 4 total sets. *Rest* no more than sixty seconds after each set.

3. **Single-arm Med Ball Carry** @30-45 seconds, followed by single-leg calf raises with feet pointing straight forward @25 repetitions.

   Please complete 4 total sets. *Rest* no more than sixty seconds after each set.

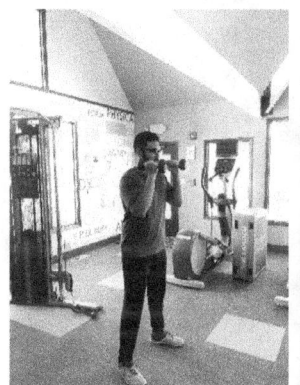 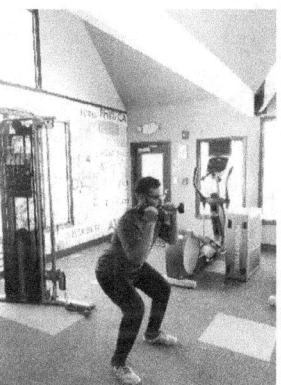 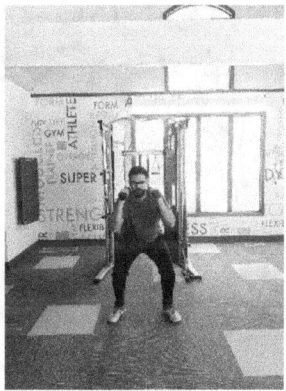

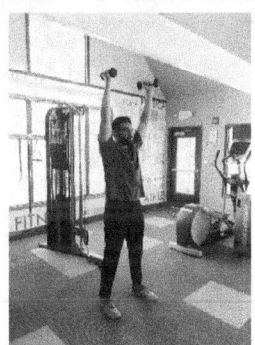 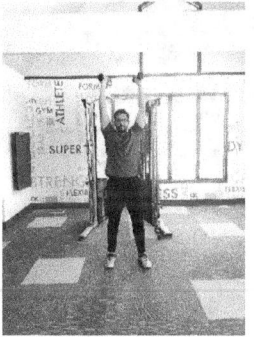

Dumbbell Thrusters 1-5

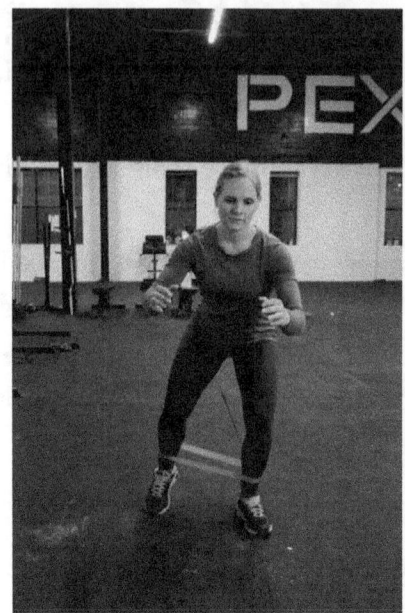 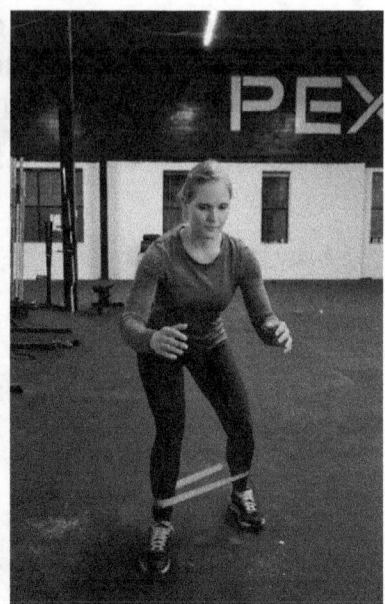

Reverse Band Walk

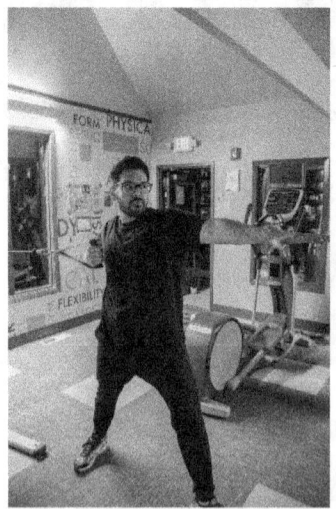 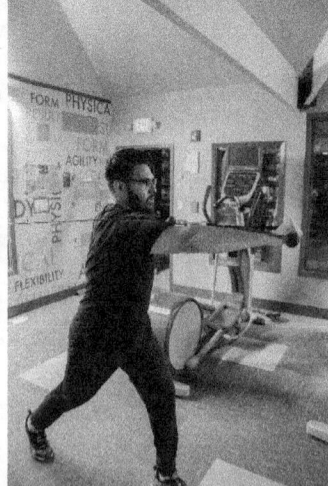

Single-arm, Split Stance, Band or Cable Press 1-2

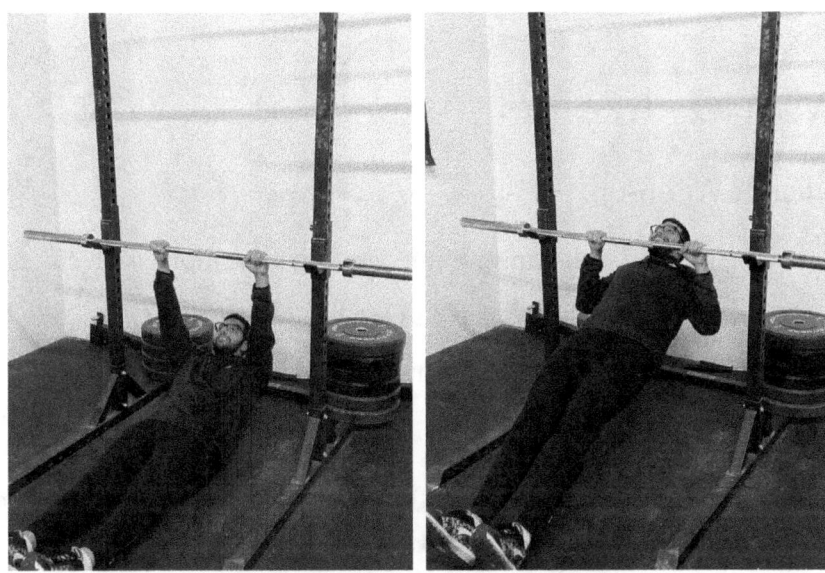

Modified Pull-up/Inverted Row
Use a smith machine if the set-up show above is not available to you

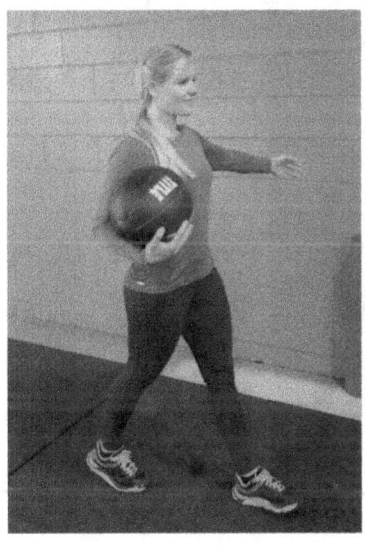

Single-arm Med Ball Carry

~Week #2~

Dynamic Warm-up:

1. T-Spine w/ Side Lunge Setup @10-15 repetitions each side.

2. 5 inchworms plus 5 World's Greatest on each side.

3. Roller on the Wall @10-15 repetitions

Session:

1. Dumbbell Front Rack Squat @10-15 reps, followed by **Single-leg RDL** @10-15 reps each side.

   Please complete 4 total sets. *Rest* no more than ninety seconds after each set.

2. Single-arm, Split Stance, Band or Cable Press @15-20 repetitions each side, followed by Modified Pull-up, i.e., inverted row @15-20 repetitions.

   Please complete 4 total sets. *Rest* no more than sixty seconds after each set.

3. Single-arm Med Ball Carry on Shoulder @30-45 seconds.

   Please complete 4 total sets. *Rest* no more than sixty seconds after each set.

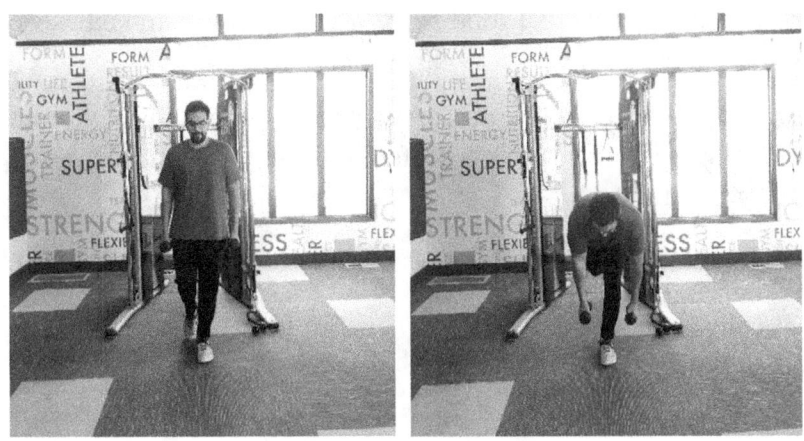

Single-leg RDL 1-2

~Week #3~

Dynamic Warm-up:

1. T-Spine w/ Side Lunge Setup @10-15 repetitions each side.

2. 5 inchworms plus World's Greatest on each side.

3. Roller on the Wall @10-15 repetitions

Session:

1. Dumbbell Thrusters @15-20 reps, followed by Reverse Band Walk @45-sixty seconds.

   Please complete 4 total sets. *Rest* no more than ninety seconds after each set.

2. Single-arm, Split Stance, Band or Cable Press @15-20 repetitions each side, followed by Modified Pull-up, i.e., inverted row @15-20 repetitions.

Please complete 4 total sets. *Rest* no more than sixty seconds after each set.

3. Single-arm Med Ball Carry @45-sixty seconds, followed by single-leg calf raises with feet pointing straight forward @25 repetitions.

Please complete 4 total sets. *Rest* no more than sixty seconds after each set.

~Week #4~

Dynamic Warm-up:

1. T-Spine w/ Side Lunge Setup @10-15 repetitions each side.

2. 5 inchworms plus 5 World's Greatest on each side.

3. Roller on the Wall @10-15 repetitions

Session:

1. Dumbbell Front Rack Squat @15-20 reps, followed by Single-leg RDL @10-15 reps each side.

Please complete 4 total sets. *Rest* no more than ninety seconds after each set.

2. Single-arm, Split Stance, Band or Cable Press @15-20 repetitions each side, followed by Modified Pull-up, i.e., inverted row @15-20 repetitions.

Please complete 4 total sets. *Rest* no more than sixty seconds after each set.

3. Single-arm Med Ball Carry on Shoulder @30-45 seconds. Please complete 4 total sets. *Rest* no more than sixty seconds after each set.

MONTH #8

WEEKS 1-4

~Week #1~

Dynamic Warm-up:

1. **Dead Bug Band Pull** with very light band @10-15 repetitions each side.
2. **Band Pull Glute Bridge** with very light band @10-15 repetitions.
3. World's Greatest @10-15 repetitions each side.

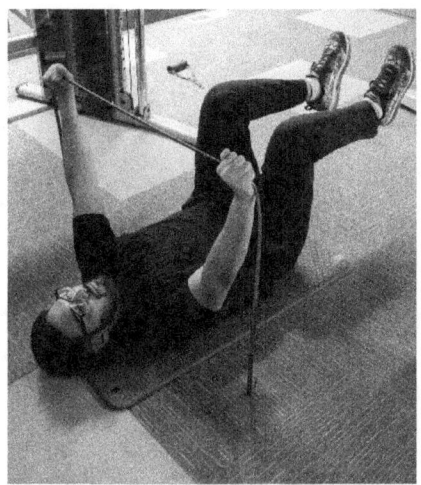 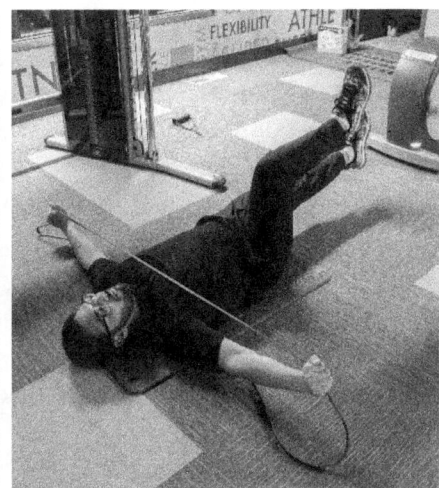

Dead Bug Band Pull 1-2

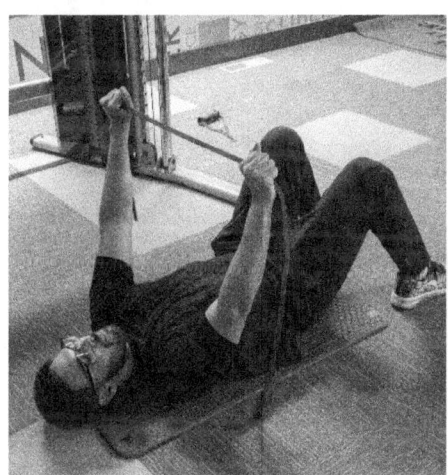 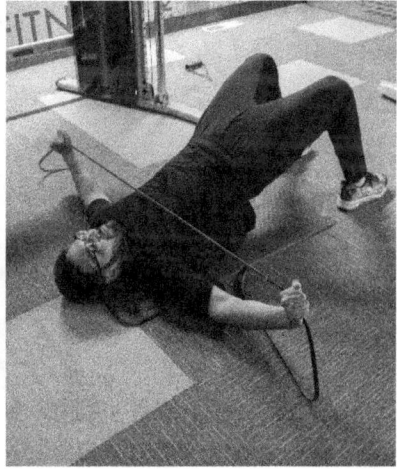

Band Pull Glute Bridge 1-2

Session:

1. **Dual Dumbbell Supinated Front Rack Squat** @10-15 reps, followed by Band or Cable Pull Through @15-20 repetitions.

   Please complete 4 total sets. *Rest* no more than ninety seconds after each set.

2. Triple Extension Cable Twists with rope attachment @10-15 repetitions each side, followed by Seated, High Cable Rope Row @15-20 repetitions.

   Please complete 4 total sets. *Rest* no more than sixty seconds after each set.

3. Standing Med Ball press to Row @15-20 repetitions, followed by **Bear Hug Med Ball Carry** @30-45 seconds.

   Please complete 4 total sets. *Rest* no more than sixty seconds after each set.

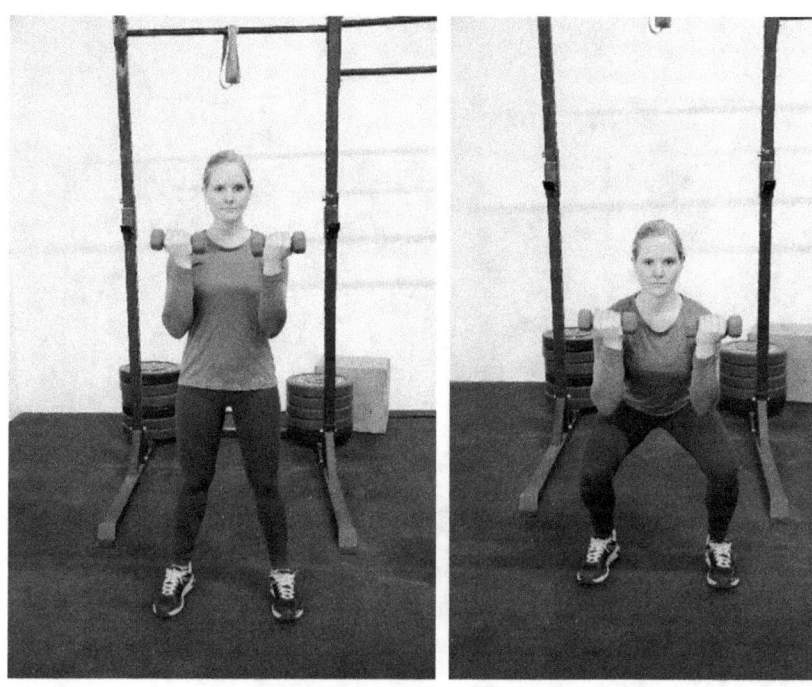

Dual Dumbbell Supinated Front Rack Squat
Be deliberate throughout this entire movement.
Go slower than normal.

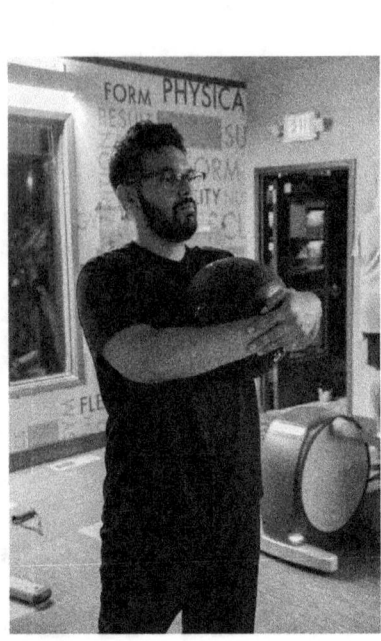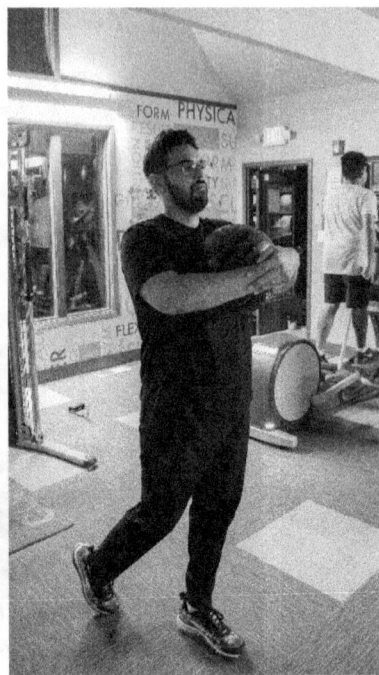

Bear Hug Med Ball Carry 1-2

~Week #2~

Dynamic Warm-up:

1. Dead Bug Band Pull with very light band @10-15 repetitions each side.

2. Band Pull Glute Bridge with very light band @10-15 repetitions

3. World's Greatest @10-15 repetitions each side.

Session:

1. **Reverse Dumbbell Goblet Squat** @10-15 reps, followed by Band or Cable Pull Through @15-20 repetitions.

   Please complete 4 total sets. *Rest* no more than ninety seconds after each set.

2. **Triple Extension Low to High with rope attachment** @10-15 repetitions each side, followed by **Air Squat Rope Row** @10-15 repetitions.

   Please complete 4 total sets. *Rest* no more than sixty seconds after each set.

3. **Standing Med Ball press to Row** @20-25 repetitions, followed by **Overhead Med Ball Carry** @30-45 seconds.

   Please complete 4 total sets. *Rest* no more than sixty seconds after each set.

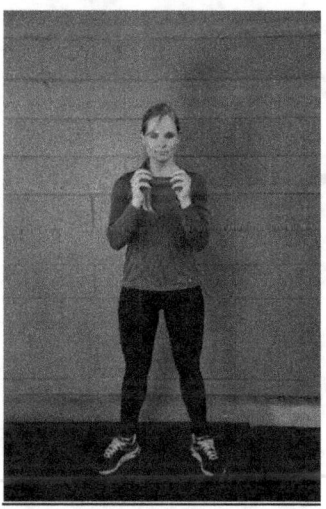

Reverse Dumbbell Goblet Squat

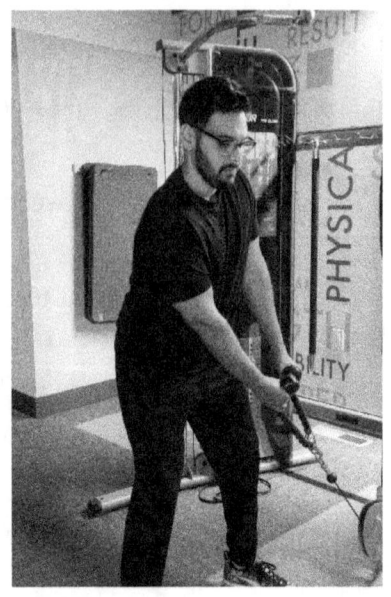 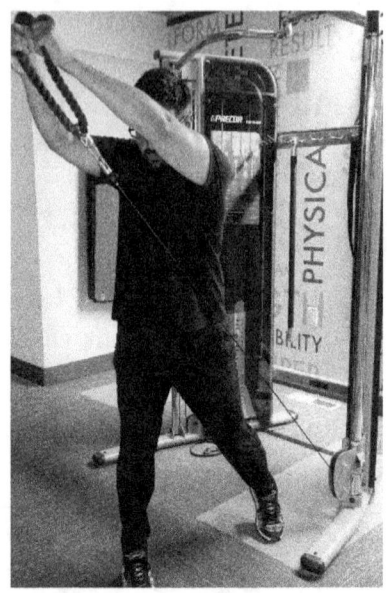

Triple Extension Low to High with rope attachment 1-2

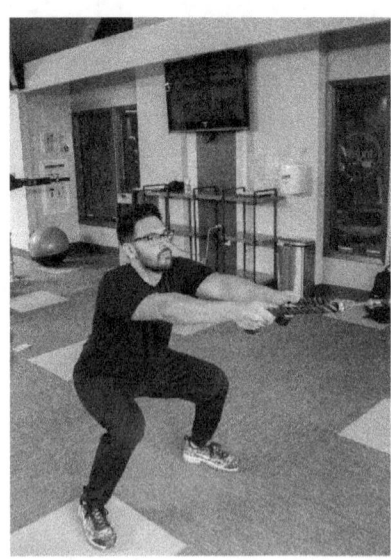 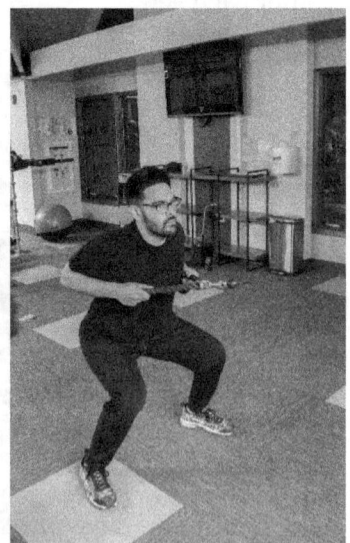

Air Squat Rope Row 1-2

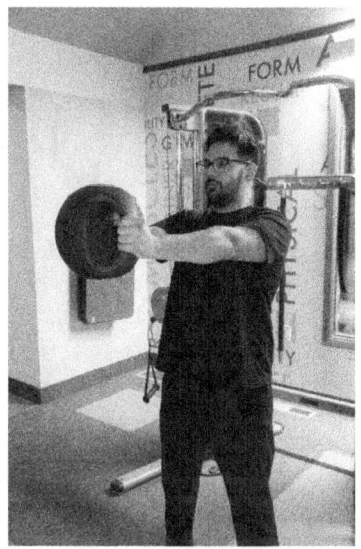 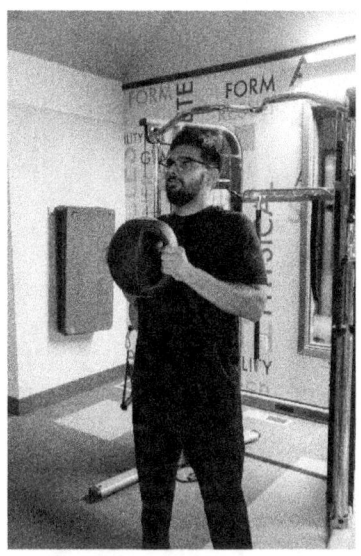

Standing Med Ball press to Row 1-2

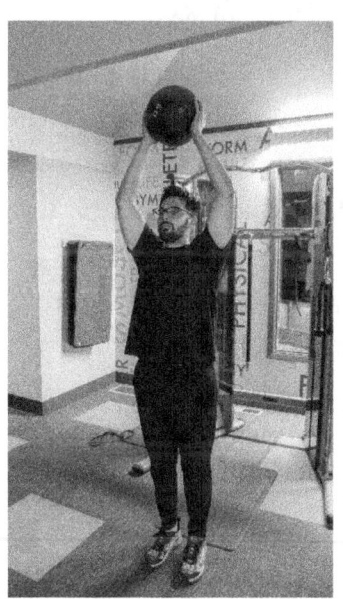 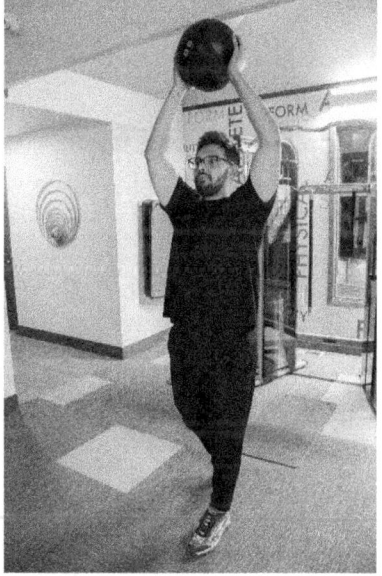

Overhead Med Ball Carry 1-2

~Week #3~

Dynamic Warm-up:

1. Dead Bug Band Pull with very light band @10-15 repetitions each side.

2. Band Pull Glute Bridge with very light band @10-15 repetitions.

3. World's Greatest @10-15 repetitions each side.

Session:

1. Dual Dumbbell Supinated Front Rack Squat @15-20 reps, followed by Band or Cable Pull Through @20-25 repetitions.

    Please complete 4 total sets. *Rest* no more than ninety seconds after each set.

2. Triple Extension Cable Twists with rope attachment @10-15 repetitions each side, followed by Seated, High Cable Rope Row @20-25 repetitions.

    Please complete 4 total sets. *Rest* no more than sixty seconds after each set.

3. Standing Med Ball press to Row @20-25 repetitions, followed by Bear Hug Med Ball Carry @45-sixty seconds.

    Please complete 4 total sets. *Rest* no more than sixty seconds after each set.

~Week #4~

Dynamic Warm-up:

1. Dead Bug Band Pull with very light band @10-15 repetitions each side.

2. Band Pull Glute Bridge with very light band @10-15 repetitions.

3. World's Greatest @10-15 repetitions each side.

Session:

1. Reverse Dumbbell Goblet Squat @15-20 reps, followed by Band or Cable Pull Through @20-25 repetitions.

   Please complete 4 total sets. *Rest* no more than ninety seconds after each set.

2. Triple Extension Low to High with rope attachment @10-15 repetitions each side, followed by Air Squat Rope Row @15-20 repetitions.

   Please complete 4 total sets. *Rest* no more than sixty seconds after each set.

3. Standing Med Ball press to Row @20-25 repetitions, followed by Overhead Med Ball Carry @forty-five to sixty seconds.

   Please complete 4 total sets. *Rest* no more than sixty seconds after each set.

MONTH #9

WEEKS 1-4

~Week #1~

Dynamic Warm-up:

1. Inchworms @20 repetitions
2. **Ape Squat and reach** @10 repetitions each side.
3. **Two Steps with Ballerina toe point** @10 points each toe

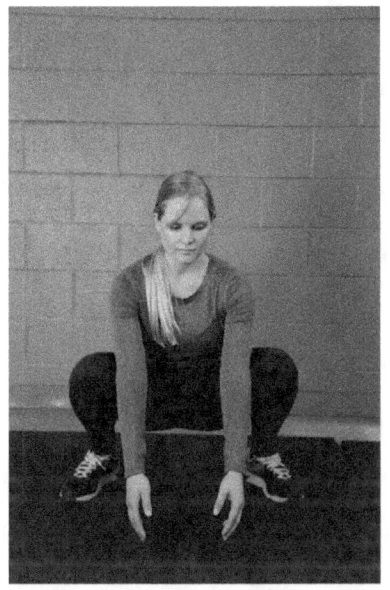 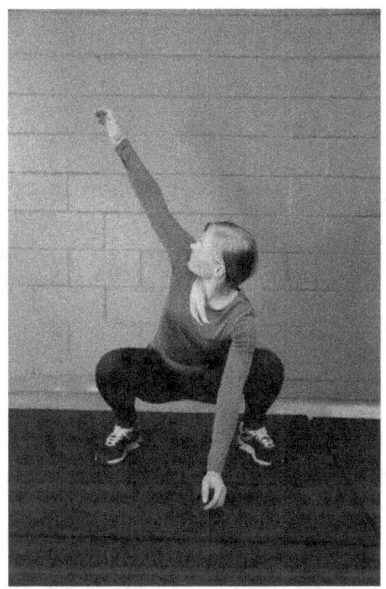

Ape Squat and reach 1-2

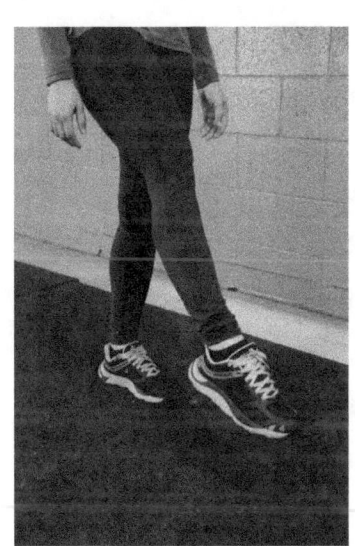 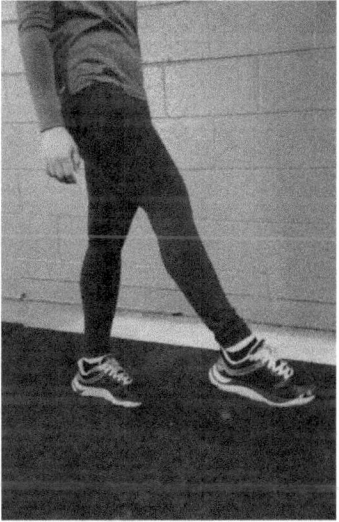

Two Steps with Ballerina Toe-Point 1-2

Session:

1. **Light Dumbbell Overhead Squat** @10-15 reps, followed by **Body-Weight Kick Throughs** @5 each side.

   Please complete 4 total sets. *Rest* no more than ninety seconds after each set.

2. **Seated High Cable Single-arm Rope Row** @15-20 repetitions each side.

   Please complete 4 total sets. *Rest* no more than sixty seconds after each set.

3. **Body-Weight Bear Crawl** @30-45 seconds.

   Please complete 4 total sets. *Rest* no more than sixty seconds after each set.

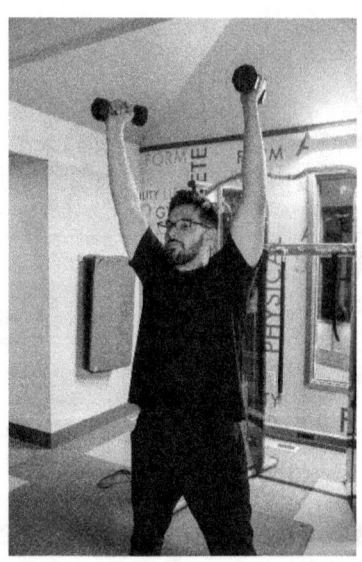

Light Dumbbell Overhead Squat

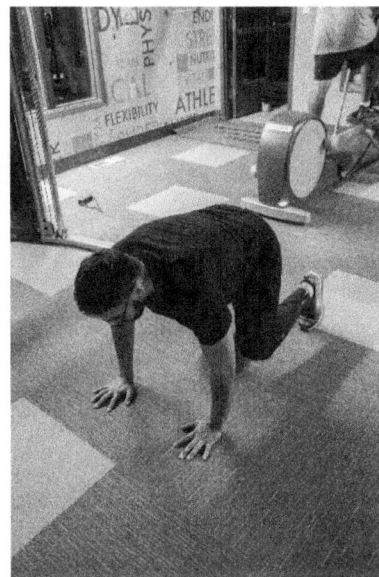 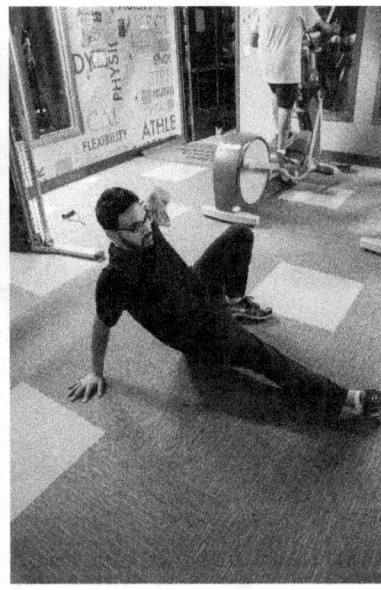

Body-Weight Kick Throughs 1-2

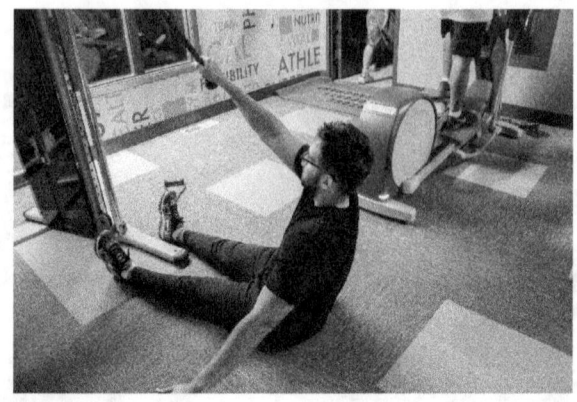

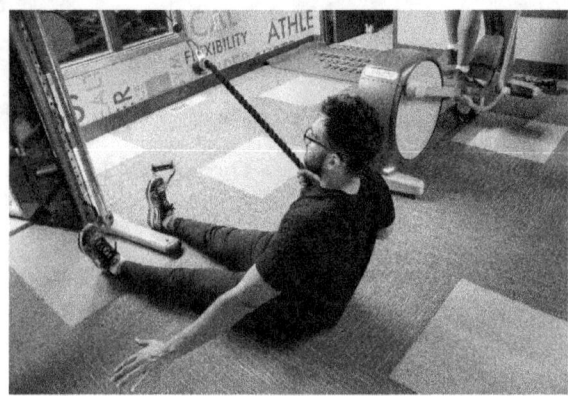

Seated High Cable, Single-arm Rope Row 1-2

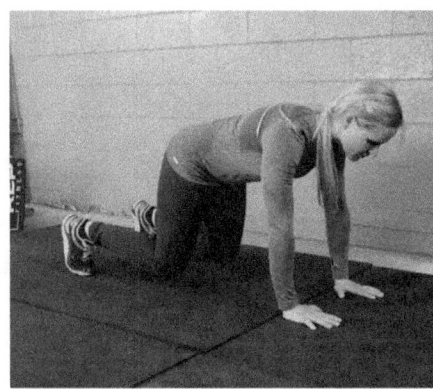
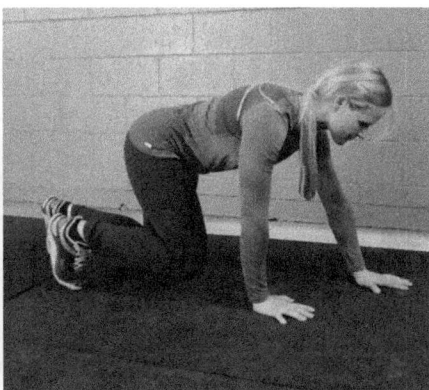
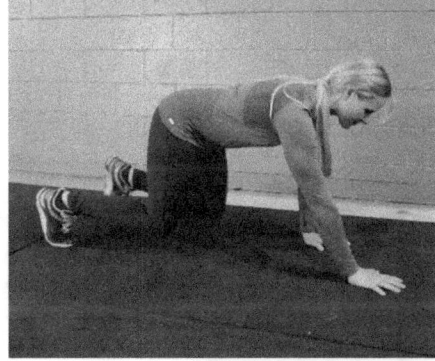
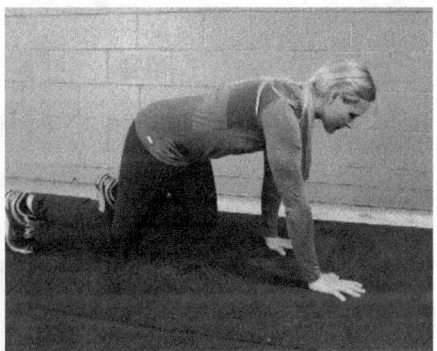
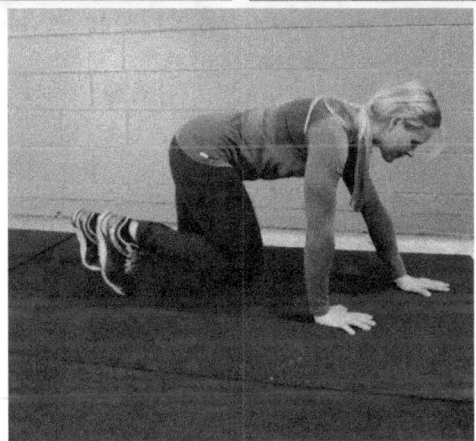

Body Weight Bear Crawl 1-5

~Week #2~

Dynamic Warm-up:

1. Inchworms @20 repetitions

2. Ape Squat and reach @10 repetitions each side.

3. Two Steps with Ballerina toe point @10 points each toe

Session:

1. Light Dumbbell Single-arm Overhead Squat @10-15 reps each side, followed by body weight kick throughs @6 each side.

   Please complete 4 total sets. *Rest* no more than ninety seconds after each set.

2. **Standing Face Pull** with rope or band @10-15 repetitions each side.

   Please complete 4 total sets. *Rest* no more than sixty seconds after each set.

3. Reverse *only* Body Weight Bear Crawl @30-45 seconds.

   Please complete 4 total sets. *Rest* no more than sixty seconds after each set.

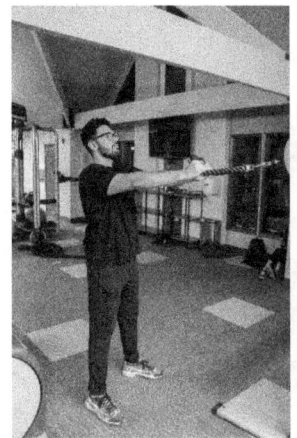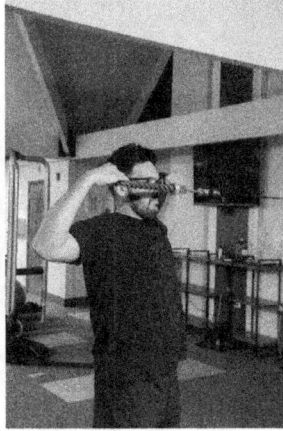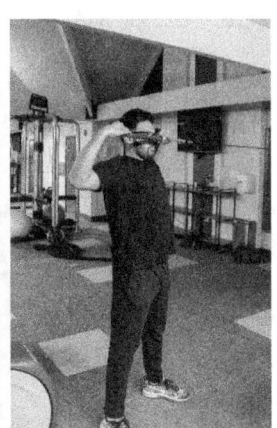

Standing Face Pull 1-3

~Week #3~

Dynamic Warm-up:

1. Inchworms @20 repetitions.

2. Ape Squat and reach @10 repetitions each side.

3. Two Steps with Ballerina toe point @10 points each toe.

Session:

1. Light Dumbbell Overhead Squat @15-20 reps, followed by body weight kick throughs @7 each side.

   Please complete 4 total sets. *Rest* no more than ninety seconds after each set.

2. Seated High Cable, single-arm Rope Row @20-25 repetitions each side.

   Please complete 4 total sets. *Rest* no more than sixty seconds after each set.

3. Body Weight Bear Crawl @45-sixty seconds.

   Please complete 4 total sets. *Rest* no more than sixty seconds after each set.

~Week #4~

Dynamic Warm-up:

1. Inchworms @20 repetitions

2. Ape Squat and reach @10 repetitions each side.

3. Two Steps with Ballerina toe point @10 points each toe

Session:

1. Light Dumbbell Single-arm Overhead Squat @15-20 reps each side, followed by body weight kick throughs @6 each side.

   Please complete 4 total sets. *Rest* no more than ninety seconds after each set.

2. Standing face pull with rope or band @15-20 repetitions each side.

   Please complete 4 total sets. *Rest* no more than sixty seconds after each set.

3. Reverse *only* Body Weight Bear Crawl @forty-five to sixty seconds. Please complete 4 total sets. *Rest* no more than sixty seconds after each set.

WELCOME TO THE FAMILY!

I WANT TO INVITE you to be a part of our ever-growing Facebook community! In this community, you will have direct access to coaching from me plus support from other like-minded individuals.

I welcome and look forward to meeting you in the community! Refer to the links below to **find us** ☺

www.fitandexpecting.com

https://m.facebook.com/fitandexpecting/

ALSO find us in Instagram here:

Instagram: @fitandexpecting.llc

###

MODIFIED MOVEMENTS

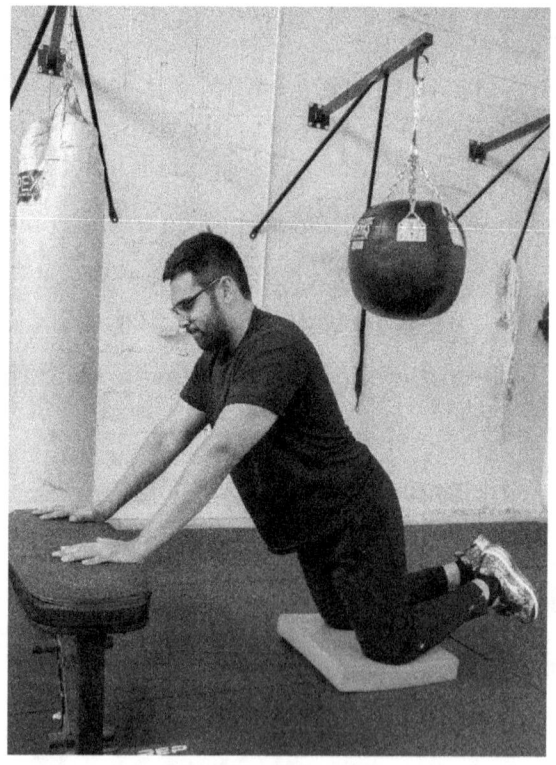

Modified Incline Pushup P1

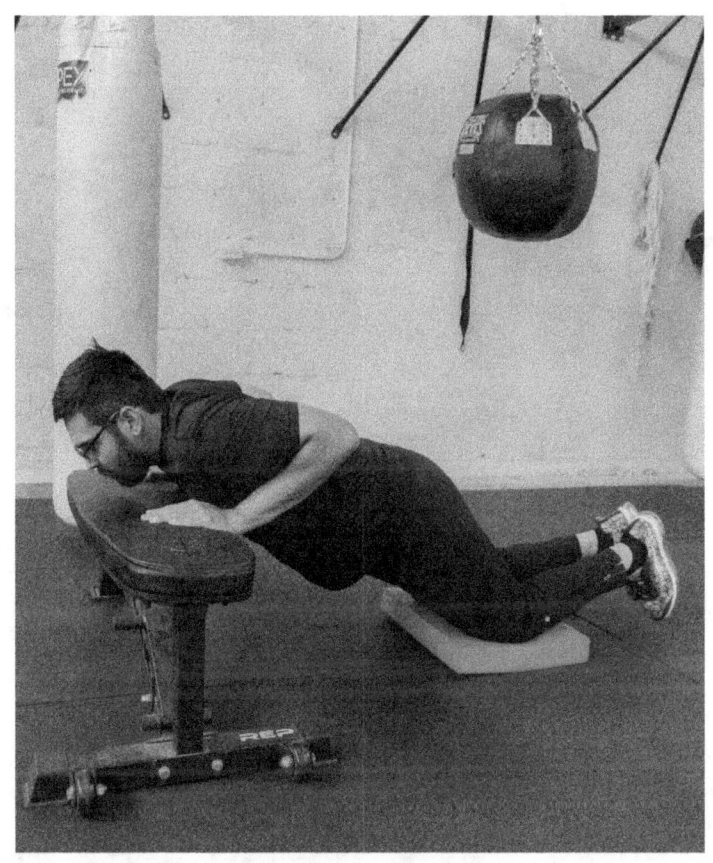

Modified Incline Pushup P2

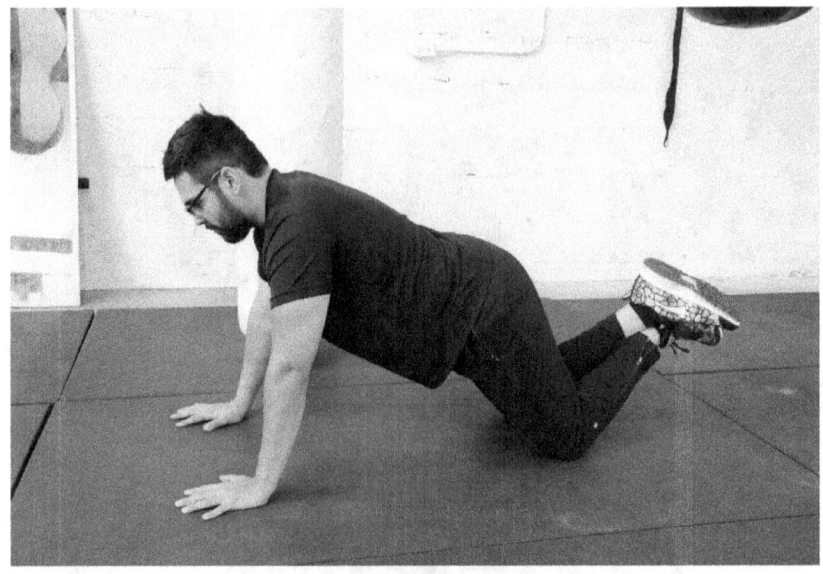

Modified Push-up 1

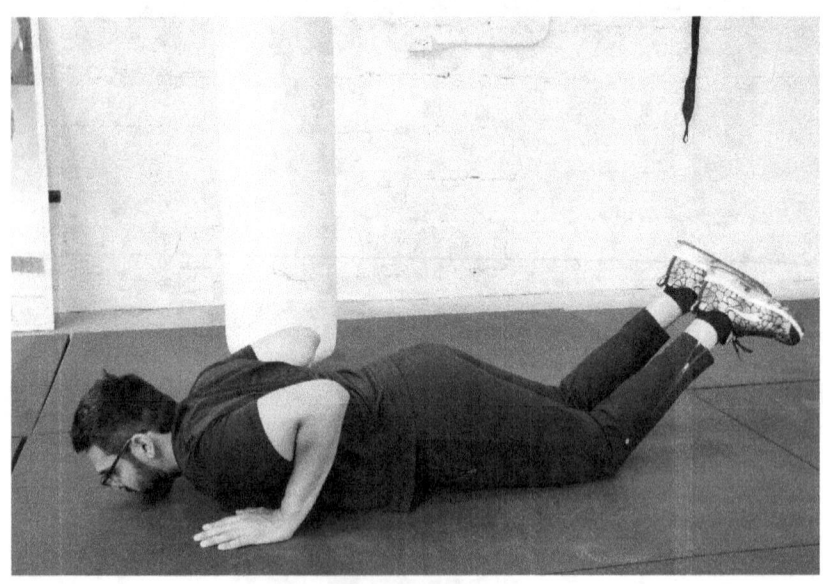

Modified Push-up 2

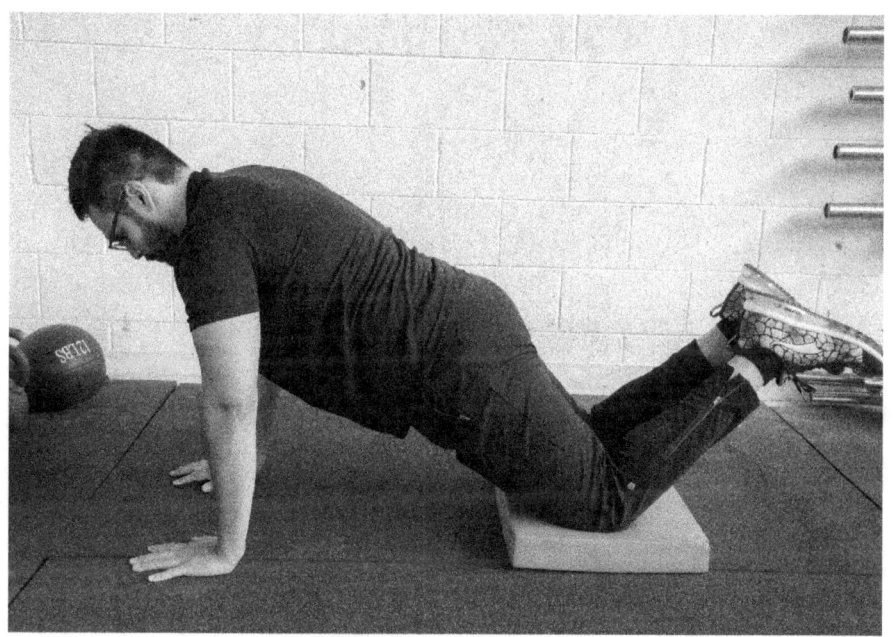

Modified Bracing Plank

ACKNOWLEDGMENTS

TO ALL THE LOVING people I have had the opportunity to lead, be led by, or watch their leadership from afar, from the bottom of my heart, I want to say thank you!

Thank you for being the catalyst and inspiration behind *Fit and Expecting*. Without you, this book would not exist!

Big love and thanks to NMC for the direction, Brennan and Aileen for the photographs, and to my family for their continuous support and belief in me.

ABOUT THE AUTHOR

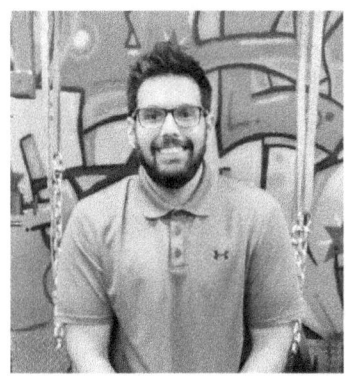

WILLIAM RAMON was born in San Antonio, Texas. He had a major turning point in his life when he lost over a hundred pounds in college. Following his transformation, he was able to compete in three full marathons, college cross-country, college golf, and the San Antonio Golden Gloves boxing tournament.

Based on his personal experiences, his first book, *The Weight Bait,* an Amazon bestseller, is an easy-to-read guide to aid readers in their quest to achieve personal bests. His book also provides the key fundamentals not only for achieving our fitness goals but to succeed at any challenge we welcome.

WILLIAM RAMON

William has a passion for golf, music, traveling, backpacking, and reading. When he is not training others, you can probably find him on the DJ decks or camping in the wilderness.

His mission is to help others find the courage to work toward their fullest potential and biggest dreams. He believes, if you have a strong foundation in health and fitness, other areas of your life will improve, too.

www.ingramcontent.com/pod-product-compliance
Lightning Source LLC
Chambersburg PA
CBHW072134280526
45788CB00002B/630